Demen

Caregiver's

Practical Guide

Manage Stress, Avoid Burnout, Find Hope, and Build Resilience

Take Care of Yourself, Manage Isolation, Your Loved One, and Financial Challenges

G.M. GRACE

First edition

Dedication

To all caregivers of dementia patients,

As I write this dedication, my heart is filled with gratitude for the incredible caregivers who have dedicated their lives to providing care and support to those suffering from dementia. Whether you work as a caregiver in a professional capacity or you're a member of a person's family providing care for a loved one, your selflessness and tireless effort have not gone unnoticed. The care and compassion you provide to those affected by dementia are invaluable. Your remarkable dedication to supporting your loved ones and delivering exceptional care despite the challenges that may arise is truly heroic. You have touched the lives of those you care for and inspired others with your kindness, patience, and selflessness. This book is dedicated to you, the caregiver. It is a tribute to your sacrifice and devotion to those in need. May your efforts be recognized, appreciated, and valued by all those whose lives you touch.

While it may never be said enough, I hope this dedication helps you realize the extent of my appreciation for all you do. May this book serve as a guide, a resource, and a support system for you. I sincerely hope that with this book in your hands, you will feel even more empowered to provide the best care possible for those suffering from dementia.

Thank you, dear reader, for dedicating your life to making the world more loving and compassionate for all those struggling with dementia. *G. M. Grace*

Index

Introduction

"One person caring about another represents life's greatest value." — Jim Rohn

Jim Rohn's quote serves as a powerful reminder of the significance and impact of caregiving, particularly in the context of dementia. Dementia is a relentless disease that progressively erodes an individual's memories, personality, and capabilities, often leaving them feeling lost and disconnected from the world around them. This journey can be arduous and heart-wrenching for the person with dementia and their caregivers.

However, amidst the challenges and emotional turmoil that dementia caregiving presents, the simple yet profound act of caring brings unparalleled meaning and value to life. By showing compassion, understanding, and support for their loved ones, caregivers forge a deep connection that transcends the barriers created by dementia. They embody the transformative power of love and dedication, proving that the human spirit can prevail even in the face of adversity.

Everything you've been told about dementia is a lie. I remember the day it happened like it was yesterday. The sun was shining through the living room window as I sat next to my mother, trying to have a conversation with her. She was looking at me, but her eyes seemed vacant. She didn't recognize me anymore. It was as if the woman who had raised me, loved me, and taught me how to be strong was no longer there.

"Mom, do you remember when we used to bake cookies together?" I asked, my voice cracking with emotion.

She stared at me, her gaze unfocused. "I... I don't know," she muttered, her voice barely above a whisper.

My heart ached as I reached for her hand, grasping it tightly. At that moment, I realized that the mother I knew was slipping away, replaced by a shell of a person that dementia had left behind. It felt as if everything I knew about dementia was wrong, and I was utterly unprepared for the journey that lay ahead.

The years that followed were filled with challenges as I cared for both my mother and my father, who eventually developed dementia as well. I had to acquire the skills to navigate the intricate journey of caregiving, encompassing tasks such as overseeing their medical needs and offering them emotional assistance.

My father's transformation was particularly surprising. I had braced myself for anger and confusion, but instead, he became gentle and loving. It was a remarkable change that served as a constant reminder that there was still a glimmer of hope amidst the darkness of dementia.

My father, once a stern and reserved man, reached out to hold my hand. His eyes were filled with warmth and love, so unlike the man I had known growing up. It was a bewildering moment, one that I would come to cherish. You see, my mother had dementia too, but her experience was vastly different. She became angry and lost the essence of who she was before the disease took hold. So, when my father's journey with dementia led him to be gentle and loving, it was a surprise, a beautifully ironic twist.

The sun was setting as we sat on the porch together, and I asked him, "Dad, can you recall when we went on a fishing trip, and you caught that enormous fish?" He looked at me, confused but smiling, and whispered, "No, but it must have been a great day." That's when it hit me: The person I knew as my father was slipping away, just like my mother had. But I realized that even though dementia was stealing their memories, it couldn't take away our love and connection in those precious moments.

Having cared for both my parents and a dear friend with dementia, I have seen firsthand the vast spectrum of experiences and emotions that dementia caregiving can bring. Through these personal experiences, coupled with my years of working in the medical field providing holistic care during the end stage of critical illnesses, I bring unique insights and perspectives to this book.

Despite the heartache and the seemingly insurmountable challenges, I discovered an ironic truth: the very thing that had robbed my parents of their personalities had also taught me the true meanings of love and resilience. It was through caring for them that I found my calling to help others in similar situations.

In the world of dementia caregiving, where days may often be filled with frustration, sorrow, and fatigue, the act of caring for another human being stands as a testament to the resilience and strength of the human heart. It is a beacon of hope that shines through the darkness, illuminating the path toward finding purpose and fulfillment in the midst of life's most daunting challenges.

As you navigate the challenging journey of dementia caregiving, I want to acknowledge and validate the numerous struggles you may be facing. In this part of our discussion, we will explore the common problems and pain points that you, as a caregiver, may encounter and offer some insight and understanding to support you during this difficult time.

First and foremost, the emotional stress that comes with caregiving is immense. Watching your loved one grapple with memory loss and cognitive decline can be heart-wrenching. The grieving process is often ongoing as you witness the person you once knew gradually change, and it's essential to allow yourself to feel and process those emotions.

Moreover, the physical demands of caregiving cannot be understated. Assisting your loved one with everyday tasks such as bathing, dressing, and feeding requires a significant amount of energy and can take a toll on your own health and well-being. It is vital to prioritize self-care and seek assistance when necessary to maintain your strength and resilience.

Financial strain is another common challenge faced by caregivers. The costs of dementia care can be staggering, particularly when it comes to professional services or specialized equipment. This added financial burden could exacerbate stress and anxiety levels, making it crucial to explore available resources and support options to help alleviate some of the financial pressure.

A lack of personal time is another obstacle that many caregivers face. Finding a balance between your personal needs and those of your loved one can be difficult, often resulting in feelings of isolation, burnout, or even resentment. To take care of yourself and keep your well-being intact, it's vital to set aside some time just for you and engage in activities that bring you joy and relaxation.

Managing difficult behaviors exhibited by individuals with dementia, such as agitation, aggression, or wandering, can be both emotionally and mentally draining. Developing patience and understanding is crucial in addressing these challenging behaviors, as well as seeking guidance and strategies from professionals or support groups.

Lastly, the uncertainty that accompanies the progressive nature of dementia can be a source of fear, anxiety, and helplessness. As your loved one's condition worsens, you may be faced with increasing levels of responsibility and decision-making. Educating yourself about dementia, connecting with others in similar situations, and seeking professional guidance can help you feel more prepared and supported as you navigate this uncertain terrain.

This journey can be unique for everyone, but the underlying motivation often comes from a place of seeking understanding, guidance, and support. I appreciate that you have chosen this resource in your quest for knowledge and assistance. I'm right here to lend you a hand in navigating the intricate world of dementia caregiving.

One of the main triggers that may have led you to this book could be the recent diagnosis of a loved one with dementia. The initial shock and confusion can be overwhelming, and the desire to understand the disease and its implications naturally drives you to seek out reliable information. In this case, you are looking for a way to make sense of the situation and prepare for the journey ahead.

Another possible catalyst is the realization that your caregiving responsibilities are increasing, and you feel ill-equipped to manage the growing demands. As your loved one's condition progresses, the need for practical advice and effective strategies to provide the best care possible becomes more urgent. This book aims to offer guidance and support as you face the challenges of dementia caregiving.

It could also be that you are experiencing emotional turmoil, stress, or burnout as a result of your caregiving role. In this case, you seek a resource that provides empathy, understanding, and reassurance, as well as practical advice on self-care and maintaining your own well-being. The content within these pages aims to help you find balance and prioritize your mental and emotional health.

Perhaps you feel isolated and alone in your caregiving journey, longing for connection and support from others who understand your struggles. This book serves as a bridge, connecting you to a community of caregivers who share your experiences and can offer valuable insights and encouragement.

Another potential catalyst is the need for guidance in making crucial decisions related to your loved one's care, such as medical interventions, living arrangements, or end-of-life planning. The weight of these decisions can be daunting, and the information in this book seeks to provide clarity and direction to help you make informed choices.

Overview

As you continue your journey through this book, get ready to explore a treasure trove of valuable insights and practical guidance to support you in your role as a dementia caregiver. While this is just an overview, it will offer you a glimpse of the shortcuts and benefits you will gain from reading further.

In the chapters ahead, you will:

1. *Gain a deeper understanding of dementia*: Develop a solid foundation of knowledge about the different types of dementia, their symptoms, and the progression of the disease. This understanding will empower you to be a more effective caregiver and advocate for your loved one.

2. *Learn how to cope with a dementia diagnosis*: Discover strategies to help you process the emotions and challenges that arise when faced with a dementia diagnosis. This knowledge will enable you to maintain resilience and strength as you navigate this new reality.

3. *Learn how to provide effective dementia care*: Acquire practical tips and tools for managing your loved one's daily needs, including personal care, communication, and maintaining a safe and

supportive environment. These skills will enhance your caregiving abilities and promote your loved one's well-being.

4. *Navigate through the challenges and pressures that come with providing dementia care:* Uncover strategies for managing the emotional and physical toll of caregiving, from dealing with difficult behaviors to addressing caregiver burnout. This guidance will help you preserve your own well-being while providing care for your loved one.

5. *Learn how to build meaningful connections:* Discover strategies to nurture and reinforce your bond with your loved one, even as dementia advances. This knowledge will enrich your caregiving experience and foster a deeper sense of connection and empathy.

6. *Find hope and grace in dementia care:* Explore the importance of cultivating a positive mindset, embracing moments of joy, and recognizing the profound value of your caregiving role. This perspective will help you find meaning and purpose in the face of adversity.

7. *Nine essential strategies for supporting your loved one:* Delve into a comprehensive list of key principles and techniques that will guide you in providing and delivering optimal care for your loved one with dementia. These strategies will serve as a

roadmap for navigating the complexities of dementia caregiving.

Throughout my many years of experience and research, I have dedicated countless hours to accumulating the knowledge and insights I now share with you in this book. Over the course of many decades, I have witnessed the journey of countless individuals and families impacted by dementia, observing both their challenges and moments of triumph. Along the way, I have also collaborated with experts in various fields and learned from their invaluable expertise.

As a dedicated caregiver myself, I have encountered the numerous challenges that dementia can present. I have felt the emotional turmoil, the frustration, and the heartache. Yet, I have also discovered the beauty in these moments, the grace in the midst of the storm, and the profound meaning of providing care to a loved one facing dementia. This personal experience has allowed me to develop a deep understanding of the complexities of dementia care, and it has been the driving force behind my mission to share this knowledge with others.

It is crucial to highlight that the wisdom shared within these pages goes beyond my personal experiences. It is the culmination of extensive research, collaboration, and valuable insights gained from professionals and caregivers alike. This book is the culmination of all those years of dedication and hard work. I hope it serves as a comprehensive guide and resource for you on your own caregiving journey.

I assure you that the time and effort invested in acquiring this knowledge has been well spent. The insights, strategies, and techniques you will discover in this book are not just theoretical concepts but practical solutions that have been tested, refined, and proven to be effective in real-life situations. These methods have been invaluable to countless caregivers who have come before you, and I am confident that they will be of immense value to you, as well.

In sharing the knowledge, I have accumulated over these many years, my primary goal is to empower and support you in providing the best possible care for your loved one. I also hope to provide you with the tools and resources you need to maintain your own well-being and resilience throughout this challenging journey.

I want to offer you a glimpse of the potential outcomes that await you. Imagine a future where you are not only equipped to provide compassionate and effective care for your loved one with dementia but are also empowered to find hope, grace, and personal growth in the process.

Once you've journeyed through this book, you'll emerge with a profound comprehension of dementia, its diverse stages, and its impact on both the individual and their loved ones. This newfound knowledge will enable you to approach your caregiving journey with greater confidence, making informed decisions about the care your loved one requires and ultimately improving their quality of life.

While you progress through the chapters, you will also learn valuable coping mechanisms to help you manage the emotional challenges that come with caring for someone with dementia. You will discover techniques to maintain your own well-being and resilience, empowering yourself to offer optimal support to your loved one while prioritizing your own well-being.

Furthermore, this book will provide practical strategies for building meaningful connections with your loved one, even as their cognitive abilities decline. You will learn how to communicate effectively, engage in activities that bring joy and comfort, and create a nurturing environment that fosters feelings of safety, belonging, and love.

The end result of your journey through this book is a transformed caregiving experience. Instead of feeling overwhelmed by the challenges of dementia care, you will be better equipped to face them head-on with a sense of purpose and optimism. Your loved one will benefit from the improved care you provide. You will discover comfort in knowing that you are making every effort to ensure their journey is filled with comfort and fulfillment to the best of your abilities.

Moreover, you will have access to a wealth of tools and resources to support your loved one throughout the various stages of dementia. The nine essential strategies outlined in this book will serve as a practical roadmap to guide you in addressing their evolving needs, ensuring they receive the utmost care at every stage of their journey.

At the end of the book, you will find a comprehensive index that includes alphabetical listings and page numbers for topics, terms, and names mentioned throughout the text.

The purpose of this index is to serve as a helpful reference tool for you, the reader. As you navigate the challenges of dementia caregiving, you may find yourself seeking specific advice, solutions, or insights related to a particular aspect of the disease or your caregiving responsibilities. The index will enable you to quickly locate and access the relevant sections of the book, ensuring that you can efficiently find the information you need when you need it.

The index covers a wide range of topics, from medical terms and symptoms to caregiving strategies, emotional support resources, and personal anecdotes. It also includes references to the names of experts, researchers, and organizations that have contributed to the field of dementia care and research. With this comprehensive approach, you can access the information that is most relevant to your specific situation and individual needs.

In addition to its practical benefits, the index also highlights the extensive research and diverse perspectives incorporated into this book. By providing a snapshot of the many topics and sources of information covered, the index underscores the book's commitment to providing you with a comprehensive and well-rounded guide to dementia caregiving.

Chapter 1:
Understanding Dementia

"To care for those who once cared for us is one of the highest honors." — Tia Walker

Dementia is a term that has, for many, been associated with a sense of dread and helplessness. The mental image of a loved one slowly losing their grip on reality, memories, and, eventually, their independence can be difficult to bear. But to truly understand and care for those afflicted with this condition, we must delve deeper into the complexities of dementia, its causes, and its progression.

At its core, dementia is not a specific disease but a collection of symptoms affecting cognitive functions, such as communication, reasoning, and memory. There are several types of dementia, each with unique characteristics and underlying causes.

The most common form is Alzheimer's disease, which accounts for an estimated 60-80% of cases. Alzheimer's is defined by the accumulation of amyloid plaques and neurofibrillary tangles in the brain, causing a gradual deterioration of brain cells.

Other prevalent types of dementia include vascular dementia, which results from impaired blood flow to the brain, often due to a stroke or series of small strokes. Lewy body dementia, another form, is marked by the presence of abnormal protein deposits called Lewy bodies in the brain, which disrupt normal functioning. Frontotemporal dementia, a less common type, affects the brain's frontal and temporal lobes and is often associated with personality and behavioral changes.

The causes of dementia can be multifaceted, with genetics, environmental factors, and lifestyle choices playing a role. For example, a family history of dementia or specific gene mutations can increase the risk of developing the condition. Head injuries, exposure to certain chemicals, and poor cardiovascular health may also contribute to the onset of dementia. Additionally, modifiable risk factors such as smoking, unhealthy diet, excessive alcohol consumption, and a sedentary lifestyle can heighten one's susceptibility to dementia.

Diagnosing dementia can be challenging due to the gradual and often subtle nature of its symptoms. Early signs may include forgetfulness, difficulty concentrating, or struggling with routine tasks. As the condition progresses, more severe symptoms emerge, such as disorientation, mood swings, and difficulty recognizing familiar faces. A comprehensive evaluation involving medical history, cognitive tests, and brain imaging is typically required to confirm a dementia diagnosis.

The progression of dementia varies greatly, depending on the severity of the condition and type, as well as the individual's overall health. Some individuals may experience a slow decline over many years, while others may deteriorate more rapidly. In some cases, the progression of dementia can be slowed or even halted through early intervention and appropriate treatments.

By understanding the intricacies of dementia, we can enhance our ability to empathize with those impacted by it and offer the essential support and care they require. One such example is the concept of "memory cafés," where people with dementia and their caregivers can socialize in a safe and welcoming environment. By fostering a sense of community and normalcy, memory cafés can alleviate some of the isolation and stigma that often accompany a dementia diagnosis.

A Closer Look at Dementia

"The only thing worse than being blind is having sight but no vision." — Helen Keller

Dementia, an umbrella term for various cognitive impairments, often steals one's vision of the future, leaving them to navigate a world that gradually fades into darkness.

By understanding the nuances of this complex condition, we can better support those affected by it and work together to minimize its impact on their lives. It's crucial to distinguish between dementia and the usual cognitive changes that occur with aging. Typical aging may involve occasional memory lapses, such as misplacing keys or struggling to recall a familiar name. However, dementia is characterized by a significant decline in cognitive functions that profoundly disrupts daily life. It's noteworthy to mention that plenty of seniors go through life without ever experiencing dementia. Dementia's incidence tends to rise as people get older, with around 6.7 million people over the age of 65 affected in 2023. Forecasts suggest that this number could escalate to roughly 14 million by 2060. Although aging is the most potent risk factor for dementia, others encompass genetic predisposition, race and Eethnicity, cardiovascular health, and traumatic brain injuries. Diagnosing dementia involves a combination of cognitive tests, physical exams, blood tests, and brain scans like CT or MRI. It is essential to identify any underlying causes and, in some cases, address reversible factors such as medication side effects, vitamin deficiencies, or thyroid hormone imbalances.

There are several common types of dementia:

1. *Alzheimer's disease*: Accounting for 60-80% of cases, Alzheimer's disease is marked by specific changes in the brain. A key symptom is difficulty remembering recent events, while issues with walking, talking, or personality changes occur later in the disease's progression.

2. *Vascular dementia*: Approximately 10% of dementia cases are linked to strokes or other blood flow issues in the brain. Symptoms depend on the affected brain area and size and typically progress in a stepwise fashion.

3. *Lewy body dementia*: People with this form of dementia may experience memory loss, movement or balance problems, changes in alertness, sleep disturbances, and visual hallucinations.

4. *Frontotemporal dementia*: This type of dementia mainly causes changes in personality and behavior due to the affected brain region. For instance, a previously cautious person may make offensive comments or neglect responsibilities.

5. *Mixed dementia*: In some cases, particularly among individuals aged 80 and older, more than one type of dementia may coexist, leading to overlapping symptoms and faster disease progression.

The treatment for dementia varies depending on the underlying cause. Neurodegenerative dementias like Alzheimer's disease currently lack a cure, but medications can aid in safeguarding the brain or managing symptoms such as anxiety or behavioral changes. Ongoing research aims to develop additional treatment options for dementia.

Types of Dementia and Their Symptoms

"It is a capital mistake to theorize before one has data." — Sherlock Holmes

Dementia, an insidious thief of cognitive abilities, presents itself in myriad forms, each with its unique characteristics and symptoms. By unraveling the mysteries of different types of dementia, we can support those affected by these neurological conditions and work towards more effective treatments.

As someone deeply interested in neurological health, I've often found myself immersed in understanding Alzheimer's disease, which is, unfortunately, the most common type of dementia. What sets this disease apart is the unusual accumulation of proteins, resulting in the creation of amyloid plaques and tau tangles scattered across the brain.

At first, the indications of Alzheimer's are quite subtle; you might notice a gentle confusion creeping in, a tendency to lose oneself in familiar surroundings, or perhaps even a habit of asking the same questions over and over again. It's easy to dismiss these signs as just simple forgetfulness, but with Alzheimer's, they could signify the beginning of a much more serious problem.

As the disease steadily advances, it takes an even heavier toll. It's heartbreaking, really, to see the impact it can have on personal relationships. Imagine struggling to recognize the faces of your loved ones or your closest friends. Imagine grappling with sudden bursts of impulsive behavior that you can't control.

The most difficult part of this journey, in my opinion, is the eventual loss of communication skills. The ability to express oneself, to share thoughts and feelings, is so central to our humanity that losing it feels like losing a part of ourselves. So, when speaking about Alzheimer's, I'm not just talking about a disease; I'm talking about a life-altering condition that affects every facet of a person's existence.

Frontotemporal dementia involves the accumulation of abnormal amounts or forms of tau and TDP-43 proteins within neurons in the frontal and temporal lobes. Symptoms can vary by type but generally include behavioral and emotional changes, movement problems, and language difficulties. Affected individuals may experience difficulty planning and organizing, impulsive behaviors, emotional flatness or excessive emotions, shaky hands, problems with balance and walking, and challenges making or understanding speech.

Lewy body dementia is marked by abnormal deposits of the alpha-synuclein protein, called "Lewy bodies," which impact the brain's chemical messengers. Cognitive decline, movement problems, sleep disorders, and visual hallucinations are common symptoms. People with this form of dementia may struggle with concentration, attention, disorganized or illogical ideas, muscle rigidity, loss of coordination, reduced facial expression, insomnia, and excessive daytime sleepiness.

Vascular dementia results from conditions, such as blood clots, that disrupt blood flow in the brain. Symptoms include forgetting current or past events, misplacing items, difficulty following instructions or learning new information, hallucinations or delusions, and poor judgment.

Accurately diagnosing dementia can be challenging, as symptoms can be similar among different types, and some people may have more than one form. Doctors typically rely on medical history, physical exams, and neurological and laboratory tests to diagnose dementia.

While there is currently no cure for these types of dementia, some treatments are available. Seeking guidance from a healthcare professional is vital to determine the most suitable approach for managing the condition.

Parkinson's disease, a progressive neurological disorder, is one type of dementia. It affects an individual's ability to move and often leads to the development of cognitive issues. In the early stages, people with Parkinson's disease dementia may struggle with reasoning and judgment, and they may hallucinate. Significantly, a distinct risk factor for dementia in individuals with Parkinson's disease is the presence of motor difficulties known as postural instability and gait disturbance (PIGD).

Creutzfeldt-Jakob disease (CJD) is an extremely rare and rapidly progressing dementia caused by the accumulation of abnormal, misfolded proteins called prions in the brain. It often leads to death within a year of diagnosis. There are three categories of CJD: sporadic, familial, and acquired. The latter, now exceedingly rare, can be caused by exposure to abnormal prion protein, primarily through the consumption of infected meat.

Wernicke-Korsakoff syndrome is a preventable and treatable type of dementia caused by a lack of vitamin B-1. This deficiency is often due to malnutrition, chronic infections, or alcoholism. People with Wernicke-Korsakoff syndrome may struggle to process information, learn new skills, and recall memory. Treatment includes hospitalization, vitamin B-1 supplementation, a balanced diet, and treatment for alcoholism if applicable.

Mixed dementia arises when an individual experiences multiple types of dementia simultaneously. The most prevalent combination involves a mixture of vascular dementia and Alzheimer's disease. Symptoms vary widely among individuals, and people with mixed dementia may experience difficulties with speech and walking as the disease progresses.

Normal pressure hydrocephalus (NPH) is a condition characterized by the buildup of excess fluid in the brain's ventricles, leading to dementia symptoms. NPH can sometimes be cured with surgery, but diagnosis often requires extensive testing to rule out other forms of dementia. Some potential causes of NPH include injury, bleeding, infection, brain tumors, and previous brain surgeries.

Huntington's disease is a genetic condition that causes dementia and manifests in two forms: juvenile-onset and adult-onset. It leads to a premature breakdown of the brain's nerve cells, resulting in impaired movement and cognitive decline. Symptoms of dementia in Huntington's disease are similar to those of other forms of dementia, with mood changes, anger, and depression particularly common. In addition to the types mentioned above, other forms of dementia include Creutzfeldt-Jakob disease, Wernicke-Korsakoff syndrome, mixed dementia, and normal pressure hydrocephalus. Each type has unique symptoms, causes, and risk factors.

Causes and Risk Factors of Dementia

The ancient Roman philosopher Seneca once wrote, "As is a tale, so is life: not how long it is, but how good it is, is what matters." This thought-provoking quote sheds light on the importance of living a good life, especially when faced with the reality of dementia and Alzheimer's disease. For millions of people worldwide, these conditions have stolen precious time and memories. By understanding these illnesses' causes and risk factors, we can take steps toward maintaining a healthy brain and possibly delaying their onset.

One of the greatest known risk factors for dementia and Alzheimer's disease is age. Although these disorders are not a normal part of aging, the risk of developing them increases with time. Most individuals diagnosed with Alzheimer's are 65 and older, with the risk doubling every five years after the age of 65. By the time a person reaches 85, the risk approaches one-third. While age is an uncontrollable factor, it is essential to recognize its impact on cognitive health.

Family history is an additional influential risk factor for dementia that remains unchangeable. Individuals with a parent, sibling, or other close relatives diagnosed with Alzheimer's are more likely to develop the disease themselves. The risk increases if multiple family members have the illness, indicating that a combination of genetic and environmental factors may be at play.

Genetics plays a significant role in Alzheimer's disease, with two categories of genes influencing its development: risk genes and deterministic genes. While deterministic genes are responsible for less than 1% of Alzheimer's cases, they directly cause the disease rather than just increasing the risk. As an author, I'm consistently fascinated by the tireless efforts of scientists in their pursuit of comprehending the part genetics play in Alzheimer's disease. Their goal? To devise personalized therapies and strategies that could revolutionize the way we manage this condition.

Beyond the unchangeable factors of age, family history, and genetics, there are other risk factors that can potentially be influenced through lifestyle choices and effective management of health conditions. One such factor is head injury, which has been linked to an increased risk of dementia. Protecting the brain from injury through measures like wearing a seatbelt, using a helmet during sports, and fall-proofing the home can help mitigate this risk.

As someone who's deeply fascinated by the intricate connection between the heart and the brain, I've come to understand the pivotal role our lifestyle choices play in shaping this relationship. It's interesting to note how conditions that harm our hearts and blood vessels, including heart disease, diabetes, strokes, hypertension, and elevated cholesterol levels, also spike the likelihood of us encountering Alzheimer's or vascular dementia.

When I started closely collaborating with my healthcare provider to keep an eye on and address any heart-related concerns, I noticed an unexpected yet welcomed side effect. My brain seemed to reap the benefits too.

Research has also indicated that strategies for overall healthy aging may contribute to a healthy brain and potentially reduce the risk of dementia and Alzheimer's. These strategies include maintaining a healthy diet, staying socially active, avoiding tobacco and excessive alcohol, and exercising both the body and mind.

Diagnosis and Progression of Dementia

The ancient philosopher Socrates once said, "An unexamined life is not worth living." This statement holds especially true when it comes to our cognitive health. Diagnosing dementia and understanding its progression can be a complex process, but the earlier it is identified, the better chance we have to manage it effectively and maintain a good quality of life.

To diagnose dementia, doctors first rule out any underlying, potentially treatable conditions that may be causing cognitive difficulties. A combination of physical exams, medical and family history, and laboratory tests help establish a comprehensive understanding of the individual's health and potential risk factors. This information serves as the foundation for further diagnostic procedures.

Cognitive and neurological tests are essential for evaluating thinking and physical functioning. These tests assess memory, problem-solving, language skills, math skills, balance, sensory response, and reflexes. By examining these aspects, healthcare professionals can determine whether an individual's cognitive abilities are consistent with dementia or another condition.

Brain scans are another crucial diagnostic tool, as they can detect strokes, tumors, and other problems that may cause dementia. Additionally, they can reveal changes in the brain's structure and function. Common types of scans include computed tomography (CT), magnetic resonance imaging (MRI), and positron emission tomography (PET).

If you or a loved one are experiencing shifts in mood or behavior, it may be beneficial to contemplate undergoing a psychiatric evaluation. This could be a vital step in understanding if these changes are stemming from depression or another mental health issue.

In certain unique instances, the use of genetic tests might be beneficial. Conducted under the watchful eyes of a medical professional and backed by the insights of a genetic counselor, these tests could potentially shed light on whether you or your loved one has specific genetic changes that could lead to certain types of dementia.

Medical professionals might also utilize cerebrospinal fluid (CSF) tests or blood tests as part of the diagnostic process for dementia. A CSF test measures the levels of proteins or other substances found in the fluid that bathes your brain and spinal cord. Blood tests, on the other hand, might be used to gauge the levels of beta-amyloid, a protein that tends to accumulate unusually in those affected by Alzheimer's disease. However, it's crucial to remember that blood test results on their own aren't definitive proof of dementia - they should be viewed as part of a comprehensive set of tests and evaluations.

Early detection of dementia symptoms is vital, as some causes can be successfully treated. While the cause of dementia is often unknown and untreatable, obtaining an early diagnosis can assist in managing the condition and planning for the future. As dementia progresses, individuals may need to adapt their daily activities and adopt new strategies to maintain their quality of life.

A primary care doctor is typically the first point of contact for individuals experiencing changes in thinking, movement, or behavior. However, specialists such as neurologists, geriatric psychiatrists, neuropsychologists, and geriatricians may also be involved in diagnosing dementia. If a specialist is not available in your community, consider contacting a medical school neurology department or a dementia clinic for expert evaluation and assistance.

Stages of Dementia

"Memory is the diary that we all carry about with us," Oscar Wilde once said. As we delve into the stages of dementia, a progressive disease that impacts memory and cognitive abilities, we must understand the devastating effects it has on the lives of those who suffer from it and their loved ones.

Dementia serves as a broad term encompassing various conditions that impact brain function, with Alzheimer's disease being the most prevalent type among them. Alzheimer's disease typically progresses through three stages: early (mild), middle (moderate), and late (severe). Each stage presents its own unique difficulties and symptoms, which may manifest differently in every individual.

In the early stage of Alzheimer's, individuals can still function independently. They may continue to work, drive, and participate in social activities. However, memory lapses become more evident, such as forgetting familiar words or misplacing everyday objects. Friends and family might notice these changes and diagnostic tools can help doctors identify symptoms. Common difficulties in this stage include struggling to find the right word or name, remembering the names of new acquaintances, difficulty performing tasks in social or work settings, and having trouble with planning or organizing.

Despite the challenges, people in the early stage of dementia can still live well by focusing on their health and wellness and engaging in meaningful activities. It is also an opportune time to establish legal, financial, and end-of-life plans, as the affected individual can actively participate in decision-making.

The middle stage of Alzheimer's is often the longest, spanning several years. As the disease advances, the affected person requires a higher level of care. During this stage, symptoms become more pronounced, causing confusion, frustration, anger, and unexpected behaviors. Nerve cell damage in the brain hinders the individual's ability to express thoughts and carry out routine tasks without assistance. Symptoms may include forgetfulness about personal history or events, moodiness, withdrawal in challenging situations, confusion about time and place, and changes in sleep patterns, among others.

At this stage, it is vital to adapt daily activities to accommodate the affected individual's needs and abilities. Caregivers might consider seeking respite care or enrolling the person in an adult daycare center to provide temporary relief from caregiving responsibilities.

In the late stage of Alzheimer's, dementia symptoms become severe, rendering the individual unable to respond to their environment, engage in conversations, or control movement. Communicating pain and discomfort is difficult, and personality changes are significant. In this stage, individuals may require round-the-clock assistance with personal care, lose awareness of their surroundings and recent experiences, and struggle with physical abilities such as walking, sitting, or swallowing. They also become more susceptible to infections, particularly pneumonia.

While the affected person may no longer initiate engagement, they can still benefit from appropriate interactions such as listening to calming music or receiving gentle touch as reassurance. In the advanced stages, caregivers may consider exploring support services such as hospice care, which prioritizes offering comfort and preserving dignity during the end-of-life phase.

How Important are the Stages of Dementia?

"Progress is impossible without change, and those who cannot change their minds cannot change anything." - George Bernard Shaw

Dementia is a multifaceted and progressive condition that impacts the brain, resulting in a gradual decline in cognitive abilities, memory, language skills, and emotional stability. Understanding the stages of dementia and how it progresses is crucial for both the individuals affected by it and their caregivers, as it provides valuable insights into the disease and how to manage it effectively.

The importance of the stages of dementia lies in their ability to help us identify the symptoms, adapt to the individual's needs, and anticipate the challenges that may arise throughout the course of the disease. It is essential to recognize that each person's journey with dementia will be unique, and the progression may not always follow a linear path. Symptoms may appear in a different order or overlap, making it difficult to place a person in a specific stage. Despite the difficulties involved, understanding the stages of dementia empowers us to provide enhanced support to individuals living with the condition, aiding them in preserving their abilities for as long as feasible. Dementia is progressive due to the nature of the brain diseases that cause it, such as Alzheimer's disease (DLB) and frontotemporal dementia (FTD). In the early stages of dementia, only a small part of the brain is damaged, causing relatively minor symptoms. However, as the disease progresses, it spreads to other parts of the brain, leading to more severe symptoms and the eventual decline of all cognitive and physical functions.

The rate at which dementia progresses varies significantly between individuals due to factors such as the type of dementia, age, and the presence of other health conditions. It is challenging to predict the progression of the disease, and some individuals may require support soon after their diagnosis, while others remain independent for several years.

To help individuals with dementia maintain their abilities for as long as possible, it is crucial to embrace a proactive approach to their well-being. Some strategies include maintaining a positive outlook, accepting support from friends, family, and professionals, engaging in physical, mental, and social activities, and ensuring proper sleep and nutrition.

Additionally, it is essential for those with dementia to manage any existing health conditions and undergo regular health check-ups to prevent new health problems from developing or worsening, which could accelerate the progression of the disease.

In cases where a person with dementia experiences a sudden change in symptoms, it is essential to consult a medical professional immediately, as it may indicate the presence of a separate health issue, such as delirium or a stroke.

Summary Box

"The only way to make sense out of change is to plunge into it, move with it, and join the dance." — Alan Watts

- Dementia is a complex, progressive condition affecting the brain, with cognitive, memory, language, and emotional decline.

  - The stages of dementia provide insights into the disease and help us anticipate challenges, adapt to individual needs, and support those living with dementia.

  - Each person's dementia journey is unique, with symptoms appearing in different orders, overlapping, or changing over time.

  - Dementia's progressive nature is due to brain diseases like Alzheimer's, vascular dementia, DLB, and FTD. As the disease progresses, it gradually spreads to other regions of the brain.

  - The rate of dementia's progression varies significantly between individuals due to factors such as the type of dementia, age, and the presence of other health conditions.

- Strategies to maintain abilities for individuals with dementia include a positive outlook, accepting support, engaging in physical, mental, and social activities, and ensuring proper sleep and nutrition.

- Regular health check-ups and managing existing health conditions are vital to prevent the progression of dementia.

- A sudden change in symptoms may indicate a separate health issue and requires immediate medical attention.

- Understanding the stages of dementia and its progression is crucial for providing tailored support, enabling those living with the condition to maintain their abilities and strive to live a fulfilling life for as long as possible.

Segue:

As we close this chapter on understanding dementia, remember the wise words of Alan Watts: "The only way to make sense out of change is to plunge into it, move with it, and join the dance." We have learned that dementia is a complex, progressive condition that affects individuals uniquely. Recognizing the stages of dementia, its progression, and strategies to maintain abilities can empower those living with the condition and their caregivers to navigate the journey with grace and resilience.

Now that we have a foundation for understanding dementia, we must face the unknown. The next chapter, "Facing the Unknown," will guide you through the emotional reactions you or your loved ones might experience, the importance of effective communication with family members and healthcare providers, and the crucial steps for planning the future and addressing legal considerations.

As we move forward, always remember that knowledge is power, and understanding the intricacies of dementia will help you adapt, grow, and make the most of every moment. So, let us continue our journey together and embrace the dance of life, even in the face of uncertainty.

Chapter 2:
Facing the Unknown

"You gain strength, courage, and confidence by every experience in which you really stop to look fear in the face. You must do the things which you think you cannot do." — Eleanor Roosevelt

Facing the Unknown: Reactions, Communication, and Planning

Life is full of uncertainties, and often we find ourselves grappling with unforeseen circumstances. It is during these times that our reactions, communication, and planning become crucial in navigating the uncharted waters ahead. In this chapter, we will probe the significance of these elements in facing the unknown, using relevant examples and insights to aid your understanding.

Reactions to the unknown can be as varied as the individuals experiencing them. Some people may feel overwhelmed, anxious, or even paralyzed by fear, while others may approach the situation with a sense of curiosity, excitement, or determination. It is essential to recognize that there is no definitive right or wrong way to respond or react; however, how we respond to uncertainty can greatly impact our ability to cope and move forward.

For instance, the COVID-19 pandemic, a global crisis beginning in 2020, took the world by storm, causing widespread panic and chaos. People's reactions ranged from fear and anxiety to denial and disbelief. Those who managed to keep a level head and adapt to the rapidly changing circumstances were better equipped to weather the storm. By acknowledging our emotions and allowing ourselves to experience them, we can better understand our reactions and develop strategies to face the unknown with courage and resilience.

Effective communication is another critical aspect of facing the unknown, especially when it comes to interacting with family, friends, and healthcare providers. Open and honest dialogue can alleviate stress, build trust, and foster a supportive environment. For example, when a family member is diagnosed with a serious illness, it is essential to have conversations about the diagnosis, treatment options, and potential outcomes. By creating a space for open dialogue, we can help each other process emotions, explore options, and make informed decisions.

In addition to honest communication, planning for the future and considering legal matters are essential steps in facing the unknown. These steps may include creating a will, establishing power of attorney, or setting up advance healthcare directives. While these topics can be uncomfortable to discuss, addressing them can provide peace of mind and ensure that our wishes are respected and carried out.

Consider the case of musician Prince, who passed away in 2016 without leaving a will. His estate, valued at over $300 million, became the subject of a lengthy and contentious legal battle among family members. This situation could have been avoided if proper planning and legal considerations had been addressed beforehand.

Your Emotions and Dementia Diagnosis

"The only way to make sense out of change is to plunge into it, move with it, and join the dance." — Alan Watts

A dementia diagnosis can evoke a whirlwind of emotions, much like a tidal wave crashing down on both the individual diagnosed and their caregivers. From relief to anger, fear, and protectiveness, the range of emotions experienced can be vast, but it is important to remember that these reactions are normal.

Supporting someone with dementia can bring up difficult feelings, and sometimes the sense of loss, grief, and worry about the future can be more disabling than the symptoms of dementia itself. It is essential to maintain connections with others and continue with daily routines, as withdrawing from these activities may worsen feelings of isolation and sadness.

Situations that can complicate feelings include being diagnosed at a younger age, worrying about employment and financial security, being in a difficult relationship, or having a type of dementia that reduces the person's ability to empathize. These situations may present additional challenges and require further support, but the crucial first step is to work through your emotions and find ways to move forward.

To cope with the myriad of emotions, consider the following strategies:

1. Let your feelings out – it is okay to cry.

2. Accept that there is no 'right' way to feel and that your feelings may change from day to day.

3. Talk about your feelings with a trained professional, such as a Certified Dementia Practitioner (CDP) or a registered nurse who specializes in dementia.

4. Write down your thoughts and feelings as a way to process and gain a better understanding of them.

Providing care for someone with dementia can be emotionally exhausting and may lead to feelings of sadness, anger, or even resentment. These emotions can be overwhelming and, if they persist, may indicate depression. Carers of people with dementia are at a much greater risk of depression, with research showing that half of all women caring for someone with dementia experience depression. It is essential to recognize these feelings and seek help from healthcare professionals, such as your GP or practice nurse, who can provide support, therapy, or medication if needed.

Preventing depression and ensuring your well-being is vital when caring for someone with dementia. Building a strong support system, planning to avoid exhaustion, practicing self-care, and seeking help with symptom management are essential steps toward a healthier, more balanced life as a caregiver. Participate in activities that bring you happiness and delight, maintain regular contact with friends and family, and prioritize your own health and well-being.

Reactions of Family and Friends to the Diagnosis

"The only way to keep a secret is to keep it to yourself. For when you tell one person, it is no longer a secret." — Mark Twain

When a loved one receives a diagnosis of dementia, it can feel like a closely guarded secret, one that can elicit a range of emotions and reactions from family and friends. In this section, we will explore the variety of responses that people may have to the news and provide guidance on how to navigate these reactions.

Many care partners find sharing the diagnosis with others can be challenging, often fearing how others will respond. The reactions of family and friends can vary greatly, which makes it essential to be prepared for diverse responses.

For some care partners, the support from their loved ones is overwhelming, with family and friends offering practical help, emotional support, and understanding. Such positive reactions can make the care partner feel loved and supported, creating a sense of unity as they face the journey ahead.

On the other hand, some family and friends may become overly protective, almost to the point of suffocating the care partner. This well-intentioned yet smothering behavior can lead to feelings of frustration and a desire for independence.

In some cases, family and friends may avoid discussing the diagnosis altogether. While this reaction may stem from discomfort or uncertainty, it can leave the care partner feeling isolated and unsupported. To bridge this communication gap, sharing information about the person with dementia's experiences can help others feel more comfortable discussing the topic. For instance, one care partner's daughter created a simple document outlining the challenges her mother was facing, which facilitated open conversations about dementia.

There are also situations where family and friends may become visibly upset upon hearing the news. Although their sadness may reflect their love and concern, it can be challenging for care partners who don't want to be pitied or treated differently.

Perhaps the most disheartening reaction is disbelief, where some family members and friends question the legitimacy of the diagnosis. This might result in a sense of exasperation, feeling unacknowledged, and the impression that others simply don't comprehend your perspective. To address this, sharing educational resources or personal experiences can help validate the diagnosis and encourage understanding.

While reactions may vary, the key to navigating them is to approach the situation with empathy and understanding. Recognizing that each person's response is shaped by their unique experiences and emotions can help care partners adapt their approach when sharing the diagnosis.

Tips for Facing Dementia in the Family

"Life can only be understood backward, but it must be lived forwards." —Søren Kierkegaard

When faced with a dementia diagnosis in the family, it's as if time itself is folding back on itself, blurring the line between the past and the present. The journey ahead can seem daunting, but with the right strategies and support, you can navigate the challenges and find meaning in the moments shared with your loved one. In this section, we will discuss some practical tips for facing dementia in the family, providing guidance on how to create an environment that fosters connection, understanding, and resilience.

1. *Allow time for adjustment:* The initial shock of the diagnosis can be overwhelming. It is essential to give yourself and your family members the space and time to process the news, mourn the future you have imagined, and accept the new reality. Be honest and open with your feelings and encourage others to do the same.

2. *Establish routines and set expectations:* Establishing a structured daily routine can offer comfort and stability to both the

individual with dementia and the caregiver. Consistent schedules and clearly defined tasks can minimize conflicts and help everyone feel more settled.

3. *Seek professional support:* An experienced dementia care counselor can provide invaluable guidance and support for both the person with dementia and their caregiver. Regular counseling sessions can help educate you about the illness, teach coping strategies, and provide emotional support.

4. *Create moments of space and respite:* As the disease progresses, mood swings and challenging behaviors may become more frequent. Giving each other space can help prevent emotional burnout and create an opportunity to regroup.

5. *Practice self-care and pacing:* Caregiving is demanding and can lead to exhaustion, stress, and even depression. Prioritize rest and self-care and be mindful of the need to physically and emotionally recharge.

6. *Incorporate daily exercise:* Regular physical activity, such as walking, can have significant benefits for the person with dementia and the caregiver. Exercise can help alleviate stress, anxiety, and depression while promoting overall well-being.

Telling Family and Friends about Dementia Diagnosis

"The most basic of all human needs is the need to understand and be understood. The best way to understand people is to listen to them." — Ralph G. Nichols

Dementia is an uninvited guest that can cause a seismic shift in the landscape of a person's life, including the way they communicate with loved ones and healthcare providers.

Yet, keeping the lines of communication open and truthful could be the secret to preserving valuable relationships and guaranteeing the finest care for someone living with dementia. In the following segment, I'd like to take you on a journey exploring how dementia can influence relationships, delve into techniques for informing others about the diagnosis, and share some handy tips for impactful communication.

1. *Telling family and friends about dementia diagnosis:* When you or a loved one is diagnosed with dementia, it's crucial to communicate openly about the situation. Share the diagnosis with family and friends and let them know about the challenges you may face, such as difficulty following conversations or remembering names. Some people may not understand dementia or may treat you differently, but

explaining your diagnosis and asking for their support can help maintain your relationships.

2. *Telling the loved one about their dementia diagnosis:* Breaking the news to the person with dementia about their diagnosis is a delicate task. Approach the conversation with empathy and care, providing information about the condition and its potential impact on their life.

3. *How relationships may change:* Dementia can change the dynamics of relationships in various ways. People with dementia may become more irritable, forget names, or require assistance with tasks they once managed independently. Moreover, the roles within the relationship may shift, with a partner or adult child becoming the primary caregiver. To navigate these changes, maintain open communication, share feelings and frustrations, and seek support from local groups and activities.

Effective communication is crucial for maintaining relationships and ensuring the well-being of the person with dementia. Here are some tips for both the person with dementia and their loved ones:

For the person with dementia:

- Inform your loved ones about your communication challenges and how they can help.

- Make eye contact and reduce distractions during conversations.

- Request that others speak more slowly and repeat information if needed.

- Ask people not to remind you that you repeat things.

For loved ones and caregivers:

- Speak clearly and slowly, using short sentences.

- Give the person with dementia time to respond and offer simple choices.

- Avoid patronizing or ridiculing their statements.

- Pay attention to body language, ensuring it is open and relaxed.

- Adapt communication methods as needed, such as rephrasing questions.

Despite the challenges dementia brings, effective communication can help maintain and even strengthen relationships. By fostering understanding, patience, and support, you can create an environment where the person with dementia and their loved ones can continue to find meaning and connection, even as the illness progresses. Remember, while dementia may alter the way we communicate, it does not erase the fundamental human need for connection and understanding.

Communicating with the Healthcare Team

The great physician and philosopher Paracelsus once said, "The art of healing comes from nature, not from the physician." In the context of dementia, the healing power of nature includes the compassion, support, and communication provided by the healthcare team, family, and friends. Establishing effective communication with healthcare providers is essential in navigating the challenges that dementia presents to both the patient and their caregivers.

Preparing for visits with healthcare professionals is vital for individuals living with dementia. A few tips to consider are documenting any changes in health, mood, memory, and behaviors, bringing a list of current prescribed medications and over-the-counter drugs, considering the presence of a care partner, family member, or friend, and making a list of questions to ask during the appointment. By being prepared and asking pertinent questions, you can ensure that the person living with dementia receives the best possible care and support.

In addition to preparing for appointments, it is important to establish a strong relationship with the healthcare team. This includes discussing the official diagnosis, understanding the tests performed, learning about potential treatments and their effects, and exploring the possibility of enrolling in clinical studies. Furthermore, it is crucial to ask about the healthcare team's familiarity with Alzheimer's disease, their roles in overseeing care, and their coordination with other members of the care team.

For caregivers, it is essential to involve the person living with dementia in all conversations regarding their care and to respect their autonomy, especially in the early stages of the disease. As the disease progresses, the care team may need to adjust to ensure proper healthcare and to maintain accurate health records.

Another factor you should consider is the insurance coverage for care planning. It's worth noting that Medicare, along with some other health insurance providers, do cover services related to care planning for folks who have recently received a diagnosis of cognitive impairment, which includes Alzheimer's and other forms of dementia.

These services can assist individuals and their caregivers in obtaining information about medical and non-medical treatments, clinical trials, and accessible community resources. Care planning is an ongoing process and should be updated at least once per year.

Planning for the Future and Legal Considerations

"The only thing we can be certain of is that nothing is certain," the famous philosopher Pliny the Elder once said. This paradoxical truth is especially relevant when considering the future of someone who has been diagnosed with dementia. Although dementia is a life-changing diagnosis, it is important to plan for the future, including legal, financial, and care considerations. This section will discuss the importance of getting started, gathering important documents, seeking professional assistance, obtaining guardianship, and considering hiring a death doula.

Getting started is crucial. Begin by thinking about long-term goals and identifying trusted family members or close friends who can provide support and be involved in planning conversations. As Alzheimer's is a progressive disease, it is vital to start having these discussions as soon as possible after a diagnosis to ensure the person living with dementia can participate in decision-making for as long as possible.

Gathering important documents is the next step. Organize and carefully review existing legal and financial documents, including copies of IDs, social security numbers, lists of medicines and doctors, Medicare cards, supplemental cards, recent bank statements, wills, life insurance statements, and receipts for burial if prepaid. These documents will guide decisions about future care and related costs. It is essential to share important passwords and the location of key documents with a trusted person in case of an emergency or unforeseen event.

Seeking professional assistance can be beneficial if the person's financial or legal situation is complex or if additional assistance is needed. A financial advisor, such as a financial planner or an estate planning attorney, can assist in identifying potential resources and devising a plan to effectively manage and preserve financial assets. A legal professional like an elder law attorney can help navigate legal decisions and documents. Many financial and legal forms can be completed without professional help, so planning ahead is attainable for every person, regardless of their financial situation.

Obtaining guardianship may be necessary when the person living with dementia is no longer able to make decisions for themselves. Guardianship is a legal process where a court appoints a responsible person or organization to manage the personal and financial affairs of a person who cannot do so independently. This can provide protection and ensure that the individual's best interests are being considered.

Considering hiring a death doula can also be helpful. A death doula, or end-of-life doula, is a non-medical professional trained to provide emotional, spiritual, and practical support to individuals and their families during the end-of-life process. They can help create a comfortable and peaceful environment, facilitate conversations about end-of-life wishes, and provide guidance on navigating the complexities of the dying process.

Care Considerations

Imagine the challenges of navigating through the fog of memory loss and confusion that come with dementia. For families and caregivers, this can be a heart-wrenching and overwhelming experience. One of the most significant decisions to make in such circumstances is determining when and how to provide long-term care for a loved one living with dementia. The process of choosing a care setting can be complex, as it involves understanding the various types of residential care, knowing when living at home is no longer an option, and asking the right questions.

Types of residential care for dementia patients vary and depend on the individual's needs. Some common options include retirement housing, assisted living, nursing homes, Alzheimer's special care units (SCUs), and life plan communities. Each type of care provides different levels of supervision, social activities, and medical assistance, thus making it crucial to evaluate the specific needs of the person living with dementia.

Retirement housing is suitable for those in the early stages of Alzheimer's who can still care for themselves independently. Assisted living closes the big gap between living independently and nursing homes by providing a comprehensive package that includes housing, meals, supportive services, and healthcare assistance. Nursing homes provide round-the-clock care and long-term medical treatment for patients with more advanced needs. Alzheimer's SCUs cater specifically to individuals with Alzheimer's and other dementias and can be found in various types of residential care communities. Life plan communities offer different levels of care based on individual needs, allowing residents to transition through various stages of care within the same community.

A time may come when the person living with Alzheimer's or dementia requires more care than can be provided at home. This realization may arise from concerns about the person's safety, the health of the caregiver or the person with dementia, or the caregiver's increasing stress and workload. In such cases, it becomes crucial to evaluate whether a residential care setting would be a better option for the individual becomes crucial.

Choosing a care setting involves careful consideration of numerous factors. When visiting different care communities, it is essential to ask questions about family involvement, staffing, programs and services, the residents, the environment, meals, and policies and procedures is essential. Inquire about staff training in dementia care, the availability of specialized services for dementia patients, and the facility's approach to handling challenging behaviors. Assess the environment for safety, comfort, and cleanliness, as well as the availability of appropriate meal options and assistance during mealtimes.

It is crucial to consider the costs associated with long-term care, as they can vary widely depending on the type of provider. Most families pay for these expenses out of their pockets, although some benefits may cover nursing care, such as long-term care insurance, Veterans benefits, and Medicaid. It is important to note that Medicare does not cover the cost of residential expenses in a care community but only covers short-term skilled care after a hospital stay.

Financial Planning

"In the midst of chaos, there is also opportunity." —Sun Tzu

When faced with a diagnosis of Alzheimer's or other dementia, financial planning can feel like navigating uncharted waters. However, being proactive and planning ahead can significantly reduce stress and help you better manage the costs that come with caring for a loved one living with dementia.

First Steps in Financial Planning

To set sail on your financial planning journey, begin with these priority steps:

1. To keep track of your financial and legal documents, create a physical worksheet or use a notebook to list all assets and debts you and your partner are responsible for. This organized approach will help you manage your financial responsibilities more efficiently.

2. Consider individuals who have a good understanding of your circumstances and those who can potentially provide support when identifying family members to be included in your financial plans.

3. Assess the costs of care, both current and future, to help you better understand the financial landscape you are navigating.

4. Review government benefits, such as assistance with prescription costs, transportation, and meals, for which you may be eligible.

5. Investigate any long-term care insurance policies you may have to determine if they can help cover future care costs.

6. Explore veterans' benefits, if applicable, as they can help with expenses.

Additionally, consider who can help you complete routine financial responsibilities, such as paying bills, arranging for benefit claims, making investment decisions, managing bank accounts, and preparing tax returns. The Consumer Financial Protection Bureau provides valuable resources to help you discuss financial responsibilities with those you trust.

Estimating Care Costs

Since Alzheimer's is a progressive disease, the type and level of care required will increase over time, and the associated costs of care will vary depending on your geographical location. To plan for your financial needs, consider costs such as:

1. Ongoing medical treatment for Alzheimer's symptoms, diagnosis, and follow-up visits.

2. Treatment or medical equipment for other medical conditions.

3. Safety-related expenses, like home safety modifications or safety services.

4. Prescription drugs.

5. Personal care supplies.

6. Adult daycare services.

7. In-home care services.

8. Full-time residential care services.

Hold a family meeting to discuss these costs and make financial plans. Utilize resources like the Managing Money: A Caregiver's Guide to Finances course to help navigate these discussions.

Navigating Financial Resources

Several financial resources may be available to help cover care costs, both now and in the future. These include:

1. Medicare, Medicare Part D, and Medigap.

2. Insurance, such as life and long-term care.

3. Employee or retirement benefits.

4. Personal assets, including savings, investments, and property.

5. Veterans' benefits.

6. Medicaid.

7. Supplemental Security Income (SSI) or Social Security Disability Insurance (SSDI) if younger than 65.

8. Community support services encompass a wide range of valuable resources, including programs such as Meals on Wheels, respite care, and transportation services. Use the Community Resource Finder to locate services in your area.

Considering Reverse Mortgages

Reverse mortgages, a form of home equity loan, enable homeowners aged 62 or older to convert a portion of their home equity into cash. While reverse mortgages do not impact Social Security or Medicare benefits, they may affect qualification for other government programs. To determine how a reverse mortgage might affect you, your beneficiaries, and your estate, consult your attorney or financial advisor.

Enlisting Professional Assistance

For those with complex financial situations or who are uncomfortable with financial planning, enlisting the help of a financial advisor, such as a financial planner or an estate planning attorney, will go a long way in getting the best financial advice.

Legal Considerations

When facing a diagnosis of dementia, or a related condition, it is crucial to address legal and financial matters as soon as possible. This is because as the disease progresses, the affected individual may lose the ability to think clearly and participate in legal and financial planning. Paradoxically, many of the legal documents required for planning must be created while the person still has the "legal capacity" to make their own decisions.

Legal capacity refers to an individual's ability to understand the consequences and implications of legal decision-making. People in the early stages of Alzheimer's or related dementia may still be able to understand many aspects of legal decision-making. Still, as the disease progresses, their decision-making abilities may deteriorate. Therefore, it is essential to act quickly and putting appropriate plans and documents in place is essential.

Legal Documents and Advance Directives

Several legal documents and advance directives can help ensure that a person's health care and financial decisions are carried out according to their wishes. These documents include the following:

1. *A Durable Power of Attorney for Health Care* is an important legal document that appoints a designated person to make healthcare decisions on behalf of an individual with dementia when they become unable to do so.

2. *Living Will:* This document records a person's wishes for medical treatment near the end of their life or if they become permanently unconscious and are unable to make decisions about emergency treatment.

3. A "*Do Not Resuscitate Order*" or DNR, as it's commonly known, is an instruction for healthcare experts not to carry out cardiopulmonary resuscitation (CPR) if an individual's heart ceases to beat or if they halt breathing. This is a directive that a doctor signs off on, and it's securely placed in the individual's medical records.

4. *Durable Power of Attorney for Finances:* This document designates an individual to make financial decisions on behalf of the person with Alzheimer's or related dementia when they are no longer capable of doing so themselves.

5. *Standard Will:* This document outlines how a person's assets and estate will be distributed among beneficiaries upon their death. It can also specify arrangements for the care of children, adult dependents, pets, gifts, trusts, and funeral and/or burial arrangements.

6. *Living Trust:* This document addresses the management of money and property while the person is still alive. A living trust appoints a trustee to hold titles to property and money on the person's behalf and provides instructions for the management of the estate.

Getting Help with Legal and Financial Planning

While healthcare providers cannot act as legal or financial advisers, they can encourage planning discussions between patients and their families. They can also guide patients, families, the care team, attorneys, and judges regarding the patient's ability to make decisions.

An elder law attorney can provide valuable assistance in interpreting state laws, devising plans for the execution of wishes, exploring financial options, and preserving financial assets. Families can seek assistance from organizations like the National Academy of Elder Law Attorneys and the American Bar Association to locate qualified attorneys. Additionally, local bar associations can help identify free legal aid options for those in need.

Geriatric care managers, who are trained social workers or nurses, can also help people with dementia and their families navigate the legal and financial planning process.

Advance Planning Advice for People with Dementia

1. Start discussions early: The rate of decline differs for each person with dementia, so involving them in planning as soon as possible is crucial.

2. Gather important papers: Make sure to store important documents in a secure location and consider providing copies to trusted family members or individuals.

3. Review plans over time: Changes in personal situations and state laws can affect legal documents, so review and update them as needed.

4. Alleviate concerns about funeral and burial arrangements: Engaging in advance planning can offer peace of mind to the person with dementia and their family.

Summary Box

"Planning is bringing the future into the present so that you can do something about it now." — Alan Lakein

In this chapter, we delved deep into the critical aspects of legal and financial planning aspects for individuals with dementia and their families. It is crucial to act promptly and make well-informed decisions to ensure a secure future is crucial. To recap the essential points discussed in this chapter:

- *Legal capacity:* Acknowledge the importance of the person's ability to comprehend and participate in legal and financial planning. Early-stage dementia patients may still understand the consequences of legal decision-making.

- *Legal documents:* Utilize various legal documents to outline healthcare and financial wishes, including advance directives, power of attorney, standard will, and living trust.

- *Advance directives:* Emphasize the significance of advance directives for healthcare and financial management, which must be prepared while the person has the legal capacity to make decisions.

- *Power of Attorney:* Designate a trustworthy individual to make healthcare and financial decisions on behalf of the person with dementia in the event that they are no longer able to make those decisions themselves.

- *Standard will:* Update the person's will to indicate how their assets and estate will be distributed upon their death and outline arrangements for the care of children, adult dependents, or pets.

- *Living trust:* Set up a living trust to manage the person's money and property while they are still alive, appointing a trustee to make financial and property decisions on their behalf.

- *Seeking professional help:* Consult with elder law attorneys, geriatric care managers, and healthcare providers to ensure proper planning and adherence to state laws.

- *Early discussions:* Initiate conversations about legal and financial planning as soon as possible after diagnosis to ensure the person with dementia can participate and make their wishes known.

- *Gather important papers:* Secure and provide copies of critical documents to family members or a trusted individual, ensuring the person's wishes are followed.

- *Review plans over time:* Reassess legal documents regularly and make updates as needed to accommodate personal situations and state law changes.

- *Protect against scams or fraud:* Implement measures to safeguard the individual's finances, such as registering for fraud alerts and placing their phone number on the National Do Not Call Registry.

- *Resources for low-income families:* Utilize available resources, such as state legal aid offices and local nonprofit agencies, for families who cannot afford legal assistance.

Segue:

In this chapter, we have journeyed through the challenging yet essential terrain of legal and financial planning for individuals with dementia and their families. By emphasizing the importance of early action, understanding legal capacity, and utilizing appropriate legal documents, we have empowered families to secure their future and protect their loved ones' best interests.

As we move forward, it is essential to remember that caring for a person with dementia is not just about addressing legal and financial matters. It is also about providing the emotional, physical, and mental support they need throughout their journey- the true essence of caregiving lies in caring with compassion.

In the upcoming chapter, "Caring with Compassion," we will delve into the heart of dementia caregiving. We will explore the basic principles and strategies to manage the behavioral   and psychological symptoms associated with dementia, as well as practical tips and resources to help you provide the best possible care for your loved one.

We will learn about the importance of effective communication, understanding the unmet needs behind behaviors, and adapting the environment to suit the person with dementia. We will also discuss how to maintain your well-being as a caregiver, a crucial aspect often overlooked in the quest to provide the best care possible.

As we transition from the complexities of legal and financial planning, let us prepare to embrace the deeply human aspect of caring for a loved one with dementia. Join us in the next chapter as we explore the essential tools and techniques to navigate the emotional landscape of caregiving and provide the support our loved ones deserve.

Legal Disclaimer

This book provides general information and discusses topics related to medicine, health, and related subjects. The content presented in this book, as well as any linked materials, should not be considered medical advice and is not intended to replace professional medical guidance.

If you or any other individual has a medical concern, it is essential to consult with a licensed physician or healthcare professional. It is important to emphasize that one should never dismiss or postpone seeking professional medical advice.

Promptly consulting with a qualified healthcare provider is essential for addressing any specific medical concerns or conditions. Consultation with a qualified healthcare provider is crucial for addressing specific medical concerns or conditions.

In case of a medical emergency, promptly contact your doctor, call emergency services (e.g., 911), or follow the appropriate emergency code in your country. The opinions expressed in this book do not represent those of any academic, hospital, practice, or other institution that may have been mentioned or linked within this book.

Leave a Review

As an independent author with a small marketing budget, reviews are my livelihood on this platform. If you are getting value from this book, I'd really appreciate it if you left your honest feedback by reviewing this book on Amazon. You can do so by scanning the QR code below. I love hearing from my readers, and I personally read every single review.

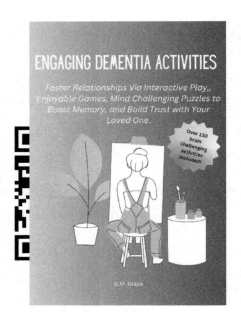

More Books by
G.M. Grace

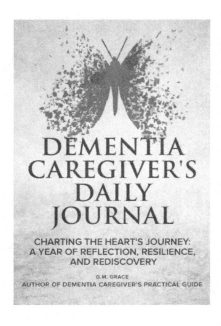

Chapter 3:
Caring with Compassion

"We rise by lifting others." — Robert Ingersoll

In the challenging journey of dementia caregiving, it's essential to remember that the quality of our care can uplift the lives of those we care for, as well as our own. As we delve into the intricacies of caregiving in this chapter, let us hold onto this guiding principle and strive to provide care with compassion and empathy.

Dementia caregiving is a delicate balance of understanding the person's individual needs, managing their symptoms, and maintaining their dignity. To navigate this complex terrain caregivers must be equipped with the right strategies and techniques to navigate this complex terrain. In this chapter, we will explore the basic principles of dementia caregiving and offer practical tips for managing behavioral and psychological symptoms.

Understanding the Person with Dementia

When caring for someone with dementia, it is crucial to see beyond their diagnosis and focus on the person they are. This means considering their personal history, preferences, values, and strengths. By doing so, you can create a care plan that honors their unique identity and fosters a sense of purpose and belonging.

For example, if the person with dementia was an avid gardener, incorporate gardening activities into their daily routine. This can help maintain a connection to their past and bring a sense of joy and accomplishment.

Communication Techniques

Effective communication is essential in dementia caregiving. As cognitive abilities decline, the person with dementia may struggle with verbal communication, leading to frustration and agitation. To overcome these challenges, caregivers should adopt supportive communication techniques, such as:

- Speaking slowly and clearly

- Using simple, direct language

- Utilizing non-verbal cues like facial expressions and gestures

- Validating their feelings and emotions

For instance, if the person with dementia becomes agitated and insists on going home when they are already at home, instead of arguing or correcting them, acknowledge their emotions and provide reassurance. You might say, "I can see you're feeling unsettled. I'm here with you, and we're safe together."

Managing Behavioral and Psychological Symptoms

As someone dealing with dementia, it's not uncommon to witness behavioral and psychological symptoms like restlessness, confrontational behavior, and a tendency to wander. These symptoms can indeed present substantial hurdles for those caring for the individual.

To effectively manage these symptoms, it is essential to identify their triggers and implement appropriate interventions. Some strategies include:

- Creating a structured, predictable routine

- Ensuring a calm, clutter-free environment

- Redirecting their attention to a more positive activity

- Offering reassurance and comfort

For example, if the person with dementia becomes agitated in the late afternoon, a phenomenon known as "sundowning," you might try engaging them in a soothing activity like listening to their favorite music or going for a gentle walk.

Self-Care for Caregivers

While caring for someone with dementia, it's vital not to neglect your own well-being. Caregiver burnout is a real and prevalent issue that can lead to adverse physical and mental health outcomes. To maintain your own health and resilience, consider the following self-care strategies:

- Seek support from family, friends, or a support group.

- Prioritize physical health through regular exercise, proper nutrition, and sufficient sleep.

- Set aside time for leisure activities and hobbies.

- Practice mindfulness and stress management techniques.

Remember that caring for yourself is not a luxury but a necessity. A healthy well-rested caregiver is better equipped to provide compassionate and effective care.

Basic Principles of Dementia Caregiving

"The greatest discovery of my generation is that human beings can alter their lives by altering their attitudes of mind." — William James

In the world of dementia care, there is a profound shift occurring towards a more person-centered approach. This shift marks a departure from the one-size-fits-all mentality of the past. It is driven by the understanding that people with dementia are still individuals with unique needs, desires, and abilities. In this section, we will discuss the seven fundamentals of effective dementia care rooted in the principles of person-centered care.

Person-Centered Care

At the core of modern dementia care lies the concept of person-centered care. It entails establishing a collaborative partnership between the caregiver, the individual with dementia, and their family members, all working together to enhance the quality of life to the best extent possible.

Joy, Comfort, Meaning, and Growth

People with dementia are capable of experiencing joy, comfort, meaning, and growth in their lives. Caregivers should focus on promoting these positive experiences by engaging individuals in activities that are meaningful and enjoyable to them. By tapping into their passions and interests, caregivers can help people with dementia find purpose and pleasure in their day-to-day lives.

Relationships

Quality of life for people with dementia depends largely on the relationships they have with their caregivers. Caregivers who take the time to build genuine connections with individuals can create a supportive and nurturing environment, which is crucial for their overall well-being.

Optimal Care within a Social Environment

Effective dementia care occurs within a social environment that fosters the development of healthy relationships between staff, family members, and residents. By creating a sense of community, caregivers can help people with dementia feel more connected and supported in their care journey.

Comprehensive Assessment and Care Planning

Good dementia care involves a thorough assessment of a person's abilities, needs, and preferences. This information is then used to create a personalized care plan, which includes strategies for addressing behavioral and communication changes, appropriate staffing patterns, and an environment that fosters community.

Uniqueness of Each Individual

Every person with dementia is unique, with a different constellation of abilities and need for support. Recognizing this individuality allows caregivers to provide care that is tailored to each person's specific circumstances, ensuring that their needs are met, and their dignity is maintained.

Knowing the Person's Life Story

Caregivers can best serve residents by learning as much as possible about their life stories, preferences, and abilities. This knowledge allows them to develop "person-centered" strategies that address the unique needs of each individual and help them feel valued and understood.

To illustrate how person-centered care can be implemented in practice, consider the following example. A caregiver discovers that a resident named Margaret was a talented painter before her dementia diagnosis. To honor her passion for art, the caregiver arranges for Margaret to participate in painting activities and even displays her artwork around the care facility. By acknowledging her love for painting, the caregiver not only engages Margaret in a meaningful activity but also helps her feel recognized and valued as an individual.

Approaches to Effectively Manage the Behavioral and Psychological Symptoms of Dementia (BPSD)

Throughout history, dementia has been a challenging and complex condition to understand and manage. It is not only a neurological issue, but also manifests in various behavioral and psychological symptoms (BPSD) that greatly impact the lives of patients and their caregivers. To effectively manage BPSD, it is crucial to identify and address the factors contributing to these symptoms, as well as to consider various non-pharmacological and pharmacological strategies for intervention.

There are several factors that may cause or contribute to BPSD, including medical, pharmacological, environmental, or social factors, and untreated pain. By identifying these underlying causes and addressing them, we can begin to alleviate the distress experienced by patients with dementia.

Understanding why a particular behavior or symptom occurs is key to managing BPSD. One way to achieve this is by gaining insight into the patient's background, including their life story, culture, religion, interests, routines, and significant life events. This can help individualize interventions and monitor the patient's response to them.

Environmental interventions, such as reducing noise, ensuring adequate lighting, providing privacy, and creating a familiar and comfortable environment, can help prevent BPSD. Behavioral interventions, including structured therapies like music therapy and cognitive-behavioral therapy, can also be beneficial in managing certain symptoms.

While non-pharmacological interventions should be prioritized, there are situations where pharmacological treatments may be necessary. However, these should be prescribed cautiously, as they are associated with serious risks and limited evidence of effectiveness. Antipsychotic medicines, for example, should only be prescribed for target symptoms or behaviors and not used as a routine method for sedation.

When thinking about the use of antipsychotic medications, it is crucial to carefully assess and balance the potential benefits against the associated risks, such as the increased risk of stroke and mortality. Close monitoring of patients receiving these medications is crucial, with the goal of reducing dosages and withdrawing treatment when possible.

Dealing with Common Dementia-Associated Behaviors

As a caregiver, dealing with common dementia-associated behaviors can be a challenging and daunting task. This section aims to provide practical strategies to help you better understand and address these behaviors while caring for your loved one with dementia. It is essential to remember that the person with dementia has a progressive brain disorder, and their personality and behavior changes are not intentional but rather a result of their condition.

1. *Wandering:* People with dementia might wander due to boredom, medication side effects, or looking for something or someone. To address wandering:

- Ensure regular exercise to minimize restlessness

- Install new locks, barriers, or monitoring systems

- Keep essential items, like coats and purses, out of sight

2. *Incontinence,* which entails the loss of control over one's bladder or bowels, can be a consequence of the progression of

dementia or due to certain external factors. Now, let's talk about how to handle incontinence:

- Establish a routine for using the toilet

- Schedule and monitor fluid intake

- Make the bathroom easily accessible and identifiable

3. *Agitation:* This refers to a range of behaviors, such as irritability, sleeplessness, or verbal/physical aggression. Agitation may be triggered by factors like environmental changes, fear, or fatigue. To handle agitation:

- Maintain a structured and familiar environment

- Minimize caffeine and sugar intake

- Offer reassurance, gentle touch, or soothing activities

4. *Repetitive speech or actions (perseveration):* People with dementia may repeat words, statements, or activities. This behavior can be triggered by anxiety, boredom, or fear. To manage repetitive speech or actions:

- Provide reassurance and comfort

- Distract the person with a snack or activity

- Avoid reminding them they just asked the same question

5. *Paranoia:* Paranoia can be a distressing symptom for both the person with dementia and the caregiver. To manage paranoia:

- Offer reassurance and validation

- Remain calm and avoid arguing

- Distract the person or change the subject

6. *Sleeplessness/sundowning:* This phenomenon often occurs late in the day, leading to agitation and confusion. To address sleeplessness/sundowning:

- Establish a bedtime routine

- Limit daytime napping

- Keep the environment calm and well-lit

7. *Eating/nutrition:* Dementia can cause changes in appetite and eating habits. To ensure proper nutrition:

- Offer small, nutritious meals frequently

- Adapt to the person's changing preferences

- Make mealtimes a social and enjoyable experience

8. *Bathing:* Bathing can be a challenging task for a person with dementia. To facilitate easier bathing:

- Maintain a familiar and comfortable routine

- Ensure safety by using non-slip mats and handrails

- Be patient and offer reassurance throughout the process

9. *UTIs (Urinary Tract Infections):* UTIs can worsen dementia symptoms, so it's essential to recognize and address them quickly. To prevent UTIs:

- Encourage regular fluid intake

- Practice proper hygiene

- Monitor for symptoms and seek medical attention if needed

10. *Additional problem areas:* Other challenging behaviors may include hallucinations or "shadowing," where the person with dementia imitates and follows the caregiver. To manage these behaviors:

- Offer verbal and physical reassurance

- Distract or redirect the person with an activity

- Involve the person in a task, like folding laundry, to make them feel useful

Handling Troubling Behavior

First and foremost, it is crucial to acknowledge that we cannot alter or change a person with dementia. Their behavior is driven by a brain disorder that has shaped who they have become. Rather than attempting to control their behavior, focus on accommodating and adapting to it. By changing our own behavior or the physical environment, we can often have a positive impact on our loved one's behavior.

One crucial aspect of managing dementia-related behaviors is recognizing that they serve a purpose. Individuals with dementia may encounter challenges in expressing their needs directly. Still, their actions often stem from an attempt to meet a need, whether it's a desire to be productive, a response to boredom, or a physical necessity like hunger or thirst.

Understanding that behaviors are triggered is another key principle in dementia care. All behaviors occur for a reason, whether due to something someone said or did or a change in the environment. The key to changing behavior is identifying and disrupting the patterns that have been created.

It is also important to accept that what works today may not work tomorrow is also important. As dementia progresses and the factors influencing behaviors change, previously effective strategies may need to be adapted or replaced altogether. Being creative and flexible in your approach to managing difficult behaviors is essential.

Support from others is invaluable in dementia care. Reach out to local support groups, organizations, and services that can provide guidance and assistance. Remember that both you and your loved one will have good and bad days, and developing strategies to cope with the difficult days is vital.

Effective communication plays a central role in caregiving for a person with dementia. By setting a positive mood, stating your message clearly, asking simple questions, listening with your ears, eyes, and heart, breaking down activities into steps, responding with affection and reassurance, and maintaining your sense of humor, you can foster a nurturing and supportive environment for your loved one.

In dealing with specific dementia-associated behaviors, such as wandering, incontinence, agitation, repetitive speech or actions, paranoia, hallucinations, sexually inappropriate behavior, and verbal outbursts, understanding the underlying causes and triggers can provide insights into how to manage them. Often, simple adjustments to the environment, routine, or communication strategies can lead to significant improvements in your loved one's behavior and overall well-being.

Finally, it is essential to remember that these behaviors are often coping mechanisms for a person with deteriorating brain function. As challenging as they may be, your loved one's actions are not intentionally malicious or hurtful. By keeping this in mind and remaining compassionate, patient, and supportive, you can help your loved one navigate the challenges of dementia with dignity and grace.

Tips for Creating a Dementia-Friendly Environment

"The best way to find yourself is to lose yourself in the service of others." — Mahatma Gandhi

Creating a dementia-friendly environment is not only about designing care environments that cater to the physical and cognitive needs of people living with dementia but also about promoting their independence, well-being, and quality of life. To accomplish this, we must integrate the Dementia Enabling Environment Principles into our approach.

1. *Unobtrusively reduce risks:* Reducing risks is essential in creating a safe environment for those with dementia. For example, installing non-slip flooring in wet areas, using

contrasting colors for different surfaces, and incorporating discreet safety features, such as hidden locks and alarms, can help prevent accidents without making the environment feel overly restrictive.

2. *Provide a human scale:* Designing spaces that are comfortable and accessible for individuals with dementia is crucial. This can be achieved by providing seating options that accommodate different mobility levels, using familiar and recognizable furniture, and ensuring the environment is not overwhelming or intimidating.

3. *Promote visual accessibility:* Visual cues play a vital role for individuals with dementia. Enhancing lighting in spaces, using contrasting colors for important objects, and incorporating clear signage can facilitate wayfinding and minimize confusion.

4. *Reduce unhelpful stimulation:* Minimizing excessive noise, clutter, and visual distractions can help create a calming atmosphere. For instance, using soothing colors on walls, avoiding busy patterns, and providing quiet spaces for relaxation can help those with dementia feel more at ease.

5. *Optimize helpful stimulation:* While it is essential to reduce unhelpful stimulation, providing positive sensory experiences

can help improve mood and cognition. Incorporating music, pleasant smells, and tactile activities can help stimulate the senses and promote engagement.

6. *Support movement and engagement:* Encouraging physical activity and social interaction is vital for maintaining overall health and well-being. This can be achieved by providing safe, accessible spaces for walking, offering a variety of activities and programs, and designing spaces that promote social interaction.

7. *Create a familiar space:* Familiarity can help those with dementia feel more secure and comfortable in their environment. Incorporating personal items, using familiar furniture, and designing spaces that resemble a typical home environment can help create a sense of familiarity.

8. *Encourage opportunities for solitude and social engagement:* Acknowledging the significance of both social interaction and moments of solitude is essential when creating dementia-friendly environments. Providing quiet areas for relaxation and reflection, as well as communal spaces for socialization, can help support a person's emotional needs.

9. *Provide links to the community:* Maintaining connections to the local community can help those with dementia feel a sense of

belonging and purpose. Incorporating community-based activities, such as outings to local parks or shops, can help foster these connections.

10. *Respond to a vision for a way of life:* Designing a dementia-friendly environment should consider the individual's preferences, values, and lifestyle. This may involve incorporating elements of the person's cultural background, providing opportunities for continued learning and growth, and adapting the environment to meet the evolving needs of the individual.

Incorporating these principles into the design of care environments can greatly enhance the quality of life for individuals living with dementia. By prioritizing safety, comfort, and familiarity, we can create spaces that not only support the physical and cognitive needs of those with dementia but also promote their emotional wellbeing and sense of identity. Ultimately, a dementia-friendly environment is one that enables people living with dementia to live their lives with dignity, purpose, and a sense of belonging.

Summary Box

"Coming together is a beginning; keeping together is progress; working together is success." — Henry Ford

- Dementia-friendly environments prioritize the physical, cognitive, and emotional needs of individuals living with dementia, promoting independence, well-being, and quality of life.

- Integrating the Dementia Enabling Environment Principles into the design of care environments is crucial for creating spaces that cater to the unique needs of those living with dementia.

- Unobtrusively reducing risks involves incorporating discreet safety features, such as non-slip flooring and contrasting colors, to create a secure environment without feeling restrictive.

- Providing a human scale ensures that spaces are comfortable and accessible, using familiar and recognizable furniture, and avoiding overwhelming or intimidating environments.

- Allowing people to see and be seen involves using well-lit spaces, contrasting colors for important items, and clear signage to aid in wayfinding and reduce confusion.

- Reducing unhelpful stimulation involves minimizing excessive noise, clutter, and visual distractions to create a calming atmosphere.

- Optimizing helpful stimulation includes providing positive sensory experiences, such as music, pleasant smells, and tactile activities, to improve mood and cognition.

- Supporting movement and engagement involves encouraging physical activity and social interaction through the provision of safe, accessible spaces for walking and a variety of activities and programs.

- Creating a familiar space helps individuals feel secure and comfortable by incorporating personal items, familiar furniture, and designing spaces that resemble a typical home environment.

- Providing opportunities to be alone or with others recognizes the need for both social interaction and solitude, offering quiet areas for relaxation and communal spaces for socialization.

- Providing links to the community fosters a sense of belonging and purpose by incorporating community-based activities, such as outings to local parks or shops.

- Responding to a vision for a way of life involves considering the individual's preferences, values, and lifestyle, incorporating cultural elements, and adapting the environment to meet the evolving needs of the individual.

• Designing dementia-friendly environments that embody these principles enhances the quality of life for individuals living with dementia, enabling them to live with dignity, purpose, and a sense of belonging.

Segue:

In the words of the ancient Greek philosopher Heraclitus, "Change is the only constant in life." As we navigate the rough waters of dementia caregiving, it is important to remember that adaptation and resilience are key.

Throughout this chapter, we have explored the significance of creating dementia-friendly environments and the various principles that should guide their design. By incorporating these principles, we can ensure that individuals living with dementia are supported in their daily lives, allowing them to maintain independence and engage meaningfully with their surroundings. We have delved into the importance of unobtrusively reducing risks, providing a human scale, optimizing helpful stimulation, and many other crucial elements that contribute to a well-rounded, dementia-friendly environment.

Nevertheless, it is crucial to acknowledge that the journey does not conclude solely with the establishment of a supportive physical environment. The next chapter, "Navigating the Rough Waters," will address the common challenges caregivers may face as they endeavor to provide the utmost care for their loved ones living with dementia. We will delve into the emotional, physical, and logistical hurdles that may arise and offer practical solutions for overcoming these obstacles.

In the coming chapter, you can expect to gain valuable insights and strategies that will help you sail smoothly through the often-stormy seas of dementia caregiving. We will provide you with tools and techniques to manage stress, foster resilience, and maintain a strong support network for both you and the person living with dementia.

By embracing the learnings from this chapter on dementia-friendly environments and equipping yourself with the knowledge from the next chapter on navigating challenges, you will be well-prepared to face the ever-changing landscape of dementia care with confidence and grace.

Chapter 4:
Navigating the Rough Waters

Please note that information about the resources mentioned in this chapter can be found on the Resource page at the end of the book.

"Burdens are many, but shoulders are strong." — Adapted Yiddish Proverb

Caring for a loved one with dementia can be a challenging and emotional journey. The rough waters of this experience are often filled with obstacles, requiring resilience, patience, and adaptability from both caregivers and their loved ones. In this chapter, we will explore the common challenges of dementia caregiving and offer guidance on how to overcome them. By understanding these hurdles and developing the necessary skills, you can be better equipped to support your loved one while also taking care of your own well-being.

One of the most significant challenges dementia caregivers faces is the emotional toll the journey takes. The progressive nature of dementia means that caregivers must often witness their loved one's decline in cognitive function, which can be painful and disheartening. This emotional strain can lead to caregiver burnout, a state of emotional, physical, and mental exhaustion that can negatively impact both the caregiver and the person receiving care. To avoid burnout, it is crucial to cultivate healthy coping mechanisms. This includes seeking support from friends, family, or support groups, engaging in self-care activities, and setting realistic expectations for both you and your loved one.

Another challenge in dementia caregiving is communication. As dementia advances, the ability of individuals with dementia to communicate their thoughts and emotions diminishes, often resulting in frustration and misunderstandings. To improve communication, caregivers can employ several strategies, such as speaking slowly and clearly, using simple words and short sentences, maintaining eye contact, and using nonverbal cues like gestures and touch. For example, if your loved one is having a challange finding the appropriate word for an object, you can employ hand gestures to aid in their comprehension or recollection of the word.

As dementia progresses, changes in behavior can also become a challenge for caregivers. These changes can include agitation, aggression, wandering, or sleep disturbances. It's important to remember that these behaviors often stem from unmet needs or frustrations. Caregivers can manage these behaviors by trying to identify the root cause, such as pain, hunger, or boredom, and addressing it accordingly. For instance, if your loved one becomes agitated in the late afternoon, a phenomenon known as "sundowning," you might try adjusting their daily routine to include more activities earlier in the day to reduce restlessness during the evening hours.

Managing the practical aspects of caregiving can be another challenge. As dementia progresses, individuals may require assistance with daily tasks such as dressing, bathing, and eating. This can be physically demanding and time-consuming, leaving caregivers feeling overwhelmed. To help navigate these rough waters, caregivers can seek assistance from professional services, such as home care or adult daycare programs, which can provide much-needed respite and support. Additionally, using adaptive equipment and modifying the home environment can make daily tasks more manageable for both the caregiver and the person with dementia.

Financial challenges are another significant aspect of dementia caregiving. The costs of medical care, home modifications, and support services can quickly add up, causing financial stress for caregivers. To alleviate this burden, it's important to explore available resources, such as government assistance programs, financial planning services, and nonprofit organizations that provide support for dementia caregivers. For example, some communities offer low-cost or sliding-scale adult daycare programs, which can provide valuable relief for caregivers while also ensuring that their loved ones are receiving appropriate care and stimulation.

Common Challenges and Stresses of Dementia Caregiving

"Caregiving often calls us to lean into love we didn't know possible." — Tia Walker

Dementia caregiving can be an incredibly rewarding experience, but it is not without its challenges and stresses. As a caregiver, you may find yourself facing both objective and subjective burdens, as well as psychological, social, physical, and financial difficulties.

It is important to understand these challenges to effectively navigate them and provide the best possible care for your loved one while also maintaining your own well-being. This section explores the typical challenges and stresses that arise in dementia caregiving and provides guidance on effective coping strategies to navigate them.

1. *Objective and Subjective Burden*

The objective burden refers to the actual time and effort required for caregiving tasks, while the subjective burden is the caregiver's perception of the burden. Both of these factors can contribute to caregiver stress and burnout. It's important to recognize and manage these burdens by seeking help when needed, setting realistic expectations, and practicing self-care. For example, you might enlist the help of family members or professional services to share caregiving responsibilities, thus reducing the objective burden.

2. *Psychological Morbidity*

Caring for someone with dementia can take a significant toll on your mental health, potentially leading to depression and anxiety. To maintain your psychological well-being, it is beneficial to seek support from friends, family, or support groups. If necessary, don't hesitate to consult a mental health professional. Engaging in activities that bring you happiness and fulfillment and relaxation, such as hobbies or exercise, can be immensely helpful in managing and alleviating stress.

3. *Social Isolation*

Dementia caregiving can be all-consuming, making it challenging to maintain a social life. To combat social isolation, make a conscious effort to stay connected with supportive family and friends, and consider joining a caregiver's support group. These connections can provide emotional support and help you share experiences, insights, and coping strategies with others in similar situations.

4. Physical Morbidity

The stress of caregiving can lead to various health issues, such as cardiovascular disease, diabetes, insomnia, and stomach ulcers. To maintain your physical health, practice good self-care habits, including regular exercise, a healthy diet, and adequate sleep. If you observe any concerning symptoms, it is important not to hesitate to consult a healthcare professional for proper evaluation and guidance.

5. Financial Difficulties

The costs associated with long-term care can place significant financial strain on caregivers. To address these challenges, explore available resources such as government assistance programs, financial planning services, and nonprofit organizations that offer support for dementia caregivers. For example, some communities provide low-cost adult daycare programs, which can offer valuable relief while ensuring appropriate care for your loved one.

6. The Toll on Care Recipients

Dementia is a progressive disease, and as it advances, the person with dementia may face various difficulties, including wandering, incontinence, agitation, and repetitive talking. By understanding these behaviors and their underlying causes, you can better anticipate and address your loved one's needs. For instance, if your loved one tends to wander, you might create a safe and secure environment to reduce the risk of accidents or injuries.

7. Learning to Cope

Developing effective coping strategies is crucial for dementia caregivers. By understanding the challenges and stresses associated with caregiving, you can proactively manage these difficulties and ensure the best possible care for your loved one. Take advantage of available resources, including support groups, educational materials, and professional services, to enhance your caregiving skills and maintain your well-being.

Don't forget, this journey isn't one you're undertaking alone, and reaching out for assistance is a mark of resilience and commitment toward ensuring the finest care for the person you love.

Common Challenges Dementia Caregivers Face

"Feelings of guilt, however, can create added stress and anxiety, which ultimately benefits neither the caregiver nor the person for whom they are caring." — Harriet Hodgson

Dealing with caregiver guilt is a common struggle for many who provide care for their loved ones. The experience of guilt can stem from various sources and often exacerbates the challenges already faced by caregivers. This section will explore the different aspects of caregiver guilt and provide strategies for coping with these feelings.

1. *Resentment of Personal Time Lost*

As a caregiver, you might grapple with feelings of bitterness due to the time you feel you've sacrificed from your personal life owing to your caregiving obligations. It's critical to accept these emotions as a natural and valid part of the process. In dealing with this, carving out some 'me time' and partaking in activities that light up your spirit and help you unwind are fundamental. Engaging in self-care is not only crucial for your mental and physical well-being but also sets the foundation for you to be a more effective caregiver.

2. *Unresolved Issues*

Sometimes, unresolved issues from the past can impact the caregiving relationship and contribute to feelings of guilt. It is essential to confront these issues and seek resolution, whether through open communication, counseling, or simply accepting the past for what it is. Addressing and processing these emotions can lead to an enhanced caregiving experience, benefiting both you and your loved one.

3. Comparing Yourself to Others

Comparing yourself to other caregivers can exacerbate feelings of guilt and inadequacy. It's crucial to recognize that every caregiving situation is unique, and comparing yourself to others is unproductive. Focus on your strengths and acknowledge the hard work you put into providing care for your loved one.

4. Knowing Placement is Inevitable

Choosing to transition a loved one into assisted living or a nursing home can often carry a heavy burden of guilt. I want you to remember that situations evolve, and what seemed like the best decision at one time might not remain the same as time progresses. Have faith in yourself that you're making the most appropriate decision for your loved one and yourself, given the circumstances at hand.

5. *Dealing with Your Own Issues*

Caregivers may also be dealing with their own personal or health problems, which can take away from caregiving responsibilities and contribute to guilt. It's essential to address these issues and seek support, whether from friends, family, or professional help. Taking care of yourself enables you to be a better caregiver for your loved one.

Coping Strategies for Caregiver Guilt:

1. Acknowledge the guilt and understand that it's a normal emotion experienced by many caregivers.

2. Focus on the bigger picture and recognize the sacrifices you are making for your loved one.

3. Accept your flaws and limitations and appreciate your strengths as a caregiver.

4. Allocate time for yourself and prioritize engaging in activities that bring you joy and relaxation.

5. Trust that you are making the best decisions for your loved one based on the current circumstances.

6. Address unresolved issues or seek professional help to improve caregiving relationships.

7. Reach out for support from family, friends, or caregiver support groups to help you work through feelings of guilt.

Dealing with Caregiver Guilt

"The greatest test of courage on earth is to bear defeat without losing heart." — Robert Green Ingersoll

Guilt is an emotion that can both motivate and hinder caregivers in their journey to provide the best possible care for their loved ones. When managed effectively, guilt can guide our actions and help us grow. In this section, we will discuss eight tips for managing caregiver guilt and transforming it into a positive force in your caregiving journey.

1. Recognize the Feeling of Guilt

To manage guilt, it is essential first to recognize and acknowledge its presence. Unaddressed guilt can gnaw at your emotional well-being, so it is crucial to confront it and understand its source.

2. Be Compassionate with Yourself

Remind yourself that feelings, including guilt, come and go like clouds in the sky. There is no right or wrong way for a caregiver to feel. By allowing yourself to experience and accept any emotion, you can lessen the grip of guilt and focus on taking positive actions.

3. Look for the Cause of the Guilt

Examine the reasons behind your guilt. Identify the discrepancies between your "Ideal You" and your current actions or situation. By understanding the root cause of your guilt, you can work towards addressing it effectively.

4. Take Action

Once you have identified the cause of your guilt, take proactive steps to address it. For example, if you feel guilty about neglecting your own needs, find ways to prioritize self-care and seek support from others to help you maintain a balanced life.

5. Change Your Behavior to Fit Your Values

If your guilt arises from actions that do not align with your values, make an effort to adjust your behavior accordingly. For instance, if you feel guilty for not sending a card to a friend in the hospital, consider buying a set of cards to have on hand for future occasions.

6. Ask for Help

Do not hesitate to reach out to friends, family, or support groups when you need assistance or a listening ear. Sharing your feelings and experiences with others can provide valuable perspectives and help alleviate feelings of guilt.

7. Revisit and Reinvent the "Ideal You"

Recognize that your past decisions were made based on the knowledge and resources available to you at the time. As you move forward, consider refining your vision of the "Ideal You" to better align with your current values and goals. This updated image can help guide your day-to-day choices and create a meaningful legacy.

8. Care for the Caregiver

It is essential to remember that taking care of yourself is a crucial aspect of being an effective caregiver. Your loved one does not expect you to be a selfless servant, and prioritizing your well-being will enable you to provide better care in the long run.

Ways to Cope with Caregiver Guilt

Caregiver Stress and Burnout: Strategies for Self-Care and Prevention

"The demands of caregiving can be exhausting and overwhelming. But there are steps you can take to rein in stress and regain a sense of balance, joy, and hope in your life." — HelpGuide.org

In the challenging role of caregiving, it is crucial to recognize the signs of caregiver stress and burnout and to implement strategies to prevent them. By understanding the impact of caregiving on one's well-being, caregivers can take steps to maintain their health and happiness while providing the best care possible for their loved ones.

What is Caregiver Burnout?

Caregiver burnout is a state of emotional, mental, and physical exhaustion caused by the ongoing demands and stresses of caregiving. Often, the person experiencing burnout feels overwhelmed and unable to effectively care for their loved one, which can lead to feelings of guilt, frustration, and even hopelessness. The long-term nature of caregiving can compound these emotions, leading to a gradual deterioration of both the caregiver's and the care recipient's well-being.

Signs and Symptoms of Caregiver Stress and Burnout

Recognizing the signs and symptoms of caregiver stress and burnout is crucial for taking action to prevent further deterioration of the situation. Common signs of caregiver stress include anxiety, depression, irritability, exhaustion, sleep difficulties, overreacting to minor issues, worsening health problems, trouble concentrating, resentment, and neglecting personal responsibilities or leisure activities. Signs of caregiver burnout may include a significant decrease in energy, frequent illness, constant exhaustion, neglect of personal needs, dissatisfaction with caregiving, difficulty relaxing, impatience, and feelings of helplessness and hopelessness.

Strategies for Preventing Caregiver Burnout

To prevent caregiver burnout, it is essential to prioritize self-care, seek help when needed, and maintain a sense of empowerment in one's caregiving role. Here are some tips for achieving these goals:

1. *Embrace acceptance:* Rather than getting entangled in the injustice of the situation or seeking a scapegoat, I encourage

you to center your energy on embracing the truth of your role as a caregiver and the hurdles it brings.

2. *Embrace your caregiving choice:* Acknowledge the reasons behind your decision to provide care and focus on the positive aspects of that choice, such as repaying a parent for their care or upholding your values.

3. *Look for the silver lining:* Consider the ways in which caregiving has made you stronger or brought you closer to your loved one or other family members.

4. *Maintain a balanced life:* Invest in activities and relationships outside of caregiving to ensure a well-rounded and fulfilling life.

5. *Focus on what you can control:* Concentrate on how you choose to react to challenges rather than stressing over factors beyond your control.

6. *Celebrate small victories:* Remind yourself that even small efforts make a difference and that the well-being and comfort of your loved one are important.

7. *Seek appreciation and support:* Turn to friends, family members, or support groups for validation and encouragement, and

remember that your loved one would likely express gratitude if they were able.

8. *Ask for help:* Share your feelings and concerns with others and seek assistance from friends, family, or respite care providers to lighten your load.

9. *Take breaks:* Carve out time to rest and engage in activities you enjoy, which will help you recharge and ultimately provide better care.

10. *Take care of your health:* Prioritize regular doctor visits, exercise, proper nutrition, relaxation techniques, and sufficient sleep to maintain your physical and mental well-being.

11. *Join a caregiver support group:* Connect with others who understand your experiences and can offer support, advice, and camaraderie.

Ways to Take Care of Yourself

Support Services and Resources for Dementia Caregivers

Caring for a loved one with dementia can be an emotionally and physically exhausting experience. Yet, as a caregiver, it is crucial to prioritize self-care in order to provide the best support possible. Here are ten essential self-care tips to help dementia caregivers maintain their well-being, even in the face of adversity.

1. *Take a break:* Respite care can be a valuable resource for caregivers, offering a temporary break from their responsibilities. Whether going to the movies, enjoying a meal with a friend, or simply spending time in nature, taking a break is essential for rejuvenating the body and the soul.

2. *Get support:* Joining a support group through organizations like the Alzheimer's Association or the Family Caregiver Alliance can provide a sense of camaraderie and understanding, as well as practical advice from others going through similar experiences. Maintaining friendships and nurturing relationships can help alleviate stress and provide a valuable support network.

3. *Practice communication and behavior skills:* Effective communication with a loved one with dementia involves using clear, short sentences and maintaining a calm tone, volume, and cadence. Nonverbal communication, such as loving gestures or smiles, can also help make the person feel calmer and less anxious.

4. *Relax:* Pursuing hobbies and interests can provide an essential escape from the demands of caregiving. Reading a book, meditating, gardening, or enjoying a massage are just a few ways to unwind and recharge.

5. *Take care of your health:* Make time for regular doctor appointments, prioritize sleep, eat well, and don't hesitate to say "no" to obligations when necessary. Ensuring your health is in check will enable you to care for your loved one.

6. *Change "guilt" to "regret":* Recognize that as a caregiver, you may face difficult decisions, but these decisions are not inherently wrong. Rather than feeling guilty, acknowledge that you are doing the best you can in a challenging situation and focus on moving forward.

7. *Forgive yourself—often:* It's natural to feel a range of emotions as a caregiver, from anger to exhaustion. Acknowledge and accept these feelings as part of the caregiving experience and remember that they don't make you a bad person or diminish your love for your family member.

8. *Laugh:* Laughter can be a powerful stress reliever. Watch a favorite comedy, share jokes with friends, or follow humorous accounts on social media to bring a little lightness to your day.

9. *Exercise:* Physical activity, such as walking, biking, or swimming, can help release tension and promote overall well-being. Make time for regular exercise to support both physical and mental health.

10. *Ask for and accept help when offered:* Don't hesitate to seek assistance with errands, chores, or caregiving decisions. Accepting help can lighten your load and provide valuable support during challenging times.

The Best Free Resources for Dementia Caregivers

The journey of a dementia caregiver can often feel like an uphill battle, filled with emotional turbulence and moments of despair. Despite the challenges, you are not alone in your fight. In fact, many resources exist to support caregivers providing care for those with dementia, and many of them are available free of charge. Let's explore some of the best free resources available to support you in this role.

First and foremost, dementia support groups are a lifeline for many caregivers. By connecting with others facing similar challenges, caregivers can find solace, understanding, and invaluable advice from those who have been in their shoes. The Alzheimer's Association, for example, offers a searchable database of support groups, making it easy to find local, in-person meetings. For those who prefer online interaction or cannot attend in-person gatherings, ALZConnected and Caregiver Nation provide virtual support communities accessible 24/7.

In moments of crisis, the Alzheimer's Association's 24/7 Helpline is an essential resource. Available around the clock, this helpline connects caregivers with master's-level clinicians and specialists, offering crisis guidance, education, information on local programs, financial and legal resources, treatment options, and care decisions. The Alzheimer's Association also has a wealth of downloadable resources to help address many questions and concerns faced by dementia caregivers.

The Family Caregiver Alliance is another valuable resource, offering a comprehensive collection of guides, tip sheets, and caregiver stories specifically tailored to those providing care for individuals with dementia. In addition, they host online support groups, allowing caregivers to connect and share their experiences with others.

The National Alliance for Caregiving is an excellent resource for all caregivers, and if you're caring for someone with dementia, you'll find their Brain Health Conversation Guide especially beneficial. This guide, crafted in partnership with the

Alzheimer's Foundation of America, is an essential instrument to navigate complex discussions around memory changes and cognitive health.

If you're a caregiver to a veteran with dementia, the U.S. Department of Veterans Affairs has a wealth of valuable information and resources about Alzheimer's disease and other dementias. They also provide services specifically designed to support both veterans and their caregivers.

The Cleveland Clinic's Healthy Brains initiative is another source of practical guidance. Offering individualized brain health assessment tools, lifestyle advice, and the latest updates in research and medicine, this interactive resource is helpful for caregivers and those living with dementia alike. It shares knowledge on how to decrease the risk of developing dementia. It provides caregiver resources, like the therapeutic influence of pets and the newest clinical trials.

The Alzheimer's Foundation of America also has a wide range of resources available for Alzheimer's caregivers. These include a free helpline, fact sheets, community classes, webinars, and much more. One of their key initiatives is the National Memory Screening Program, which has screened over 5 million people across the U.S. so far.

The Caregiver Action Network's Family Caregiver Toolbox is yet another treasure trove of resources for caregivers. Although not exclusively dedicated to dementia care, the toolbox is packed with information and resources that any caregiver, including those caring for individuals with Alzheimer's, can find useful.

Lastly, Dementia Friendly America, a national network of communities, organizations, and individuals dedicated to supporting people living with dementia and their caregivers, provides a comprehensive list of resources and toolkits. Whether you're a caregiver or someone who wishes to advocate in your local community, they've got you covered.

Memory Cafés, which can be found in hospitals, libraries, senior centers, and other locations, provide support for those with dementia and their caregivers in a social setting. The Memory Café Directory lists hundreds of such cafés throughout the U.S.

The federal government also offers reliable resources on Alzheimer's disease and related dementias, including tips for caregivers, home safety, and caregiver health. These resources, provided by various governmental agencies such as the National Institute on Aging, the Administration for Community Living, and the U.S. Department of Veterans Affairs, offer information, support,` and encouragement for caregivers,

Summary Box

- Dementia caregiving can be an emotionally challenging and isolating journey, but numerous free resources are available to provide support and guidance.

- Dementia support groups, both in-person and online, provide caregivers with the opportunity to connect with others who share similar experiences. These groups foster a sense of community and understanding, offering a valuable support network.

- The Alzheimer's Association's 24/7 Helpline offers crisis guidance, education, and information on local programs, financial and legal resources, treatment options, and care decisions.

- The Family Caregiver Alliance and the National Alliance for Caregiving provide comprehensive resources, guides, tip sheets, and support groups tailored for dementia caregivers.

- For veteran caregivers, the U.S. Department of Veterans Affairs offers resources and services specifically designed for veterans with dementia and their caregivers.

- The Cleveland Clinic's Healthy Brains initiative provides brain health assessment tools, lifestyle tips, and up-to-date news on research and medicine for both caregivers and those living with dementia.

- The Alzheimer's Foundation of America offers a wide array of resources, including a free helpline, fact sheets, community classes, webinars, and a National Memory Screening Program.

- The Caregiver Action Network's Family Caregiver Toolbox offers helpful tips and information on all aspects of caregiving, including resources for Alzheimer's caregivers.

- Dementia Friendly America is a national network that offers resources, toolkits, and advocacy support for caregivers and those with dementia.

- Memory Cafés provide social support and combat isolation for those with dementia and their caregivers in various community settings.

- Federal government agencies, such as the National Institute on Aging and the Administration for Community Living, offer reliable resources and support for dementia caregivers, including tips for caregiver health, home safety, and navigating long-term care.

Segue:

As we draw this chapter to a close, it is essential to reflect on the critical takeaways and the significance of the resources available for dementia caregivers. Remember, you are not alone on this challenging journey. Support groups, helplines, and various organizations offer invaluable guidance, information, and assistance to help you navigate the complexities of dementia care. These resources empower you to provide the best possible care for your loved one while also taking care of your own well-being.

The paradox of dementia caregiving is that, while it can often feel isolating, there is a wealth of support available to connect you with others who share your experiences. By seeking out these resources and engaging in supportive communities, you can build resilience and develop the skills needed to face the challenges of caregiving.

As we move on to the next chapter, "Connecting Through the Fog," we will delve deeper into the importance of building meaningful connections with those with dementia. We will explore creative approaches to engage and communicate effectively with your loved one, despite the cognitive barriers dementia presents. By honing your communication skills and employing innovative strategies, you can forge stronger bonds and improve the quality of life for both you and your loved one with dementia. So, stay curious and engaged as we journey further into the world of dementia caregiving and help you navigate the fog of this complex condition.

Chapter 5:
Connecting Through the Fog

"Never believe that a few caring people can't change the world. For, indeed, that's all who ever have." — Margaret Mead

Importance of Social and Emotional Connections For People with Dementia

There was an elderly woman named Emily I had the privilege of knowing. Emily, a vibrant lady in her prime, was a social butterfly. She had the most infectious laughter and an uncanny ability to make anyone feel like the most important person in the room. As she aged, however, Emily was diagnosed with dementia. As her memory started to fade, the person who was once the life of every party started retreating into her shell.

But something remarkable happened when her family and friends came together to ensure she didn't lose the precious social connections that had always been a part of her life. Despite her condition, they found ways to engage Emily, taking her to gatherings, and encouraging interactions, even when it was challenging. They saw that these social and emotional connections were not just essential but a lifeline for Emily.

Why are these connections so important, you might ask?

Think of the brain as a muscle that needs to be exercised, just like the muscles in our bodies. Engaging with other people helps keep the brain active, maintain memory, and manage emotions. For Emily, her weekly card games with friends, albeit her ability to remember the rules was waning, served as a workout for her brain. She would laugh, engage, and for those moments, she was the Emily of the old times. Studies have shown that such socialization can even slow the progress of cognitive impairment in some cases.

For individuals with dementia, maintaining focus can often become a challenge. They might feel disoriented about their location or the time period they're in. This unsettling feeling can be mitigated through socialization. When Emily was surrounded by her loved ones, recounting tales of their shared past, it provided her with an anchor to the here and now. It gave her a sense of groundedness, making it easier to carry out everyday tasks.

But more than anything, social and emotional connections help create a feeling of inclusion. Humans, by nature, are social creatures. We thrive on relationships for stimulation and survival. For a person with dementia, this need doesn't change, but their ability to fulfill it does. For Emily, the efforts made by her family and friends to keep her involved made her feel included, loved, and cherished, despite her struggles.

Now, I'm not saying it was easy. The journey had its bumps. But Emily's family and friends found that the efforts they made were rewarded in the most heartwarming ways. They saw glimpses of the Emily they knew, the Emily who loved being around people, who laughed freely and brought joy to those around her.

The Importance of Social Interaction for Individuals with Dementia

There's an old saying that goes, "No man is an island." This age-old proverb resonates more with me now than ever before, especially as I reflect on the journey with my own father, who was living with dementia. I remember the stark difference in his demeanor when we began to incorporate more social activities into his daily routine. The transformation was a testament to the power of human connection and the importance of social interaction.

I am writing this to you because I know you, too, are on this journey with a loved one. You might be wondering how you can make a difference; help slow down the progression of dementia and bring some joy and meaning to your loved one's life. The answer lies in something as simple yet profound as social interaction.

Research shows that social interaction can decrease anxiety and agitation, increase the quality of life, and may even slow down the development of dementia. It's a startling revelation, but it makes sense. Think about it. As humans, we thrive on connection. It fuels our spirit and mind, providing a sense of purpose and belonging.

Imagine an elderly woman; let's call her Mrs. Jones. She used to be an active participant in her community, loved by her peers. But with the onset of dementia, she starts withdrawing, not out of choice, but out of fear and confusion. Her friends begin to fade away, and the vibrant woman who once thrived in the company of others now spends her days alone. This isolation can lead to a faster cognitive decline. A study involving over 2,000 elderly women found that those with a larger social network were 26% less likely to develop dementia. In Mrs. Jones's case, maintaining her social connections could have a profound impact on slowing down the progression of her disease.

Think about your loved one. Are they becoming more isolated? The power to change this lies in your hands.

Social interaction isn't just about warding off loneliness; it's also about mental stimulation, which has tangible physical benefits. Remember how we used to feel after a lively discussion at the dinner table or a heartwarming chat with a dear friend? It's not just our hearts that are lifted; our brains also benefit from these engagements.

Consider Mr. Brown, a retired schoolteacher diagnosed with dementia. Before his diagnosis, he used to love spending time with his former students, discussing everything from current events to classic literature. Once he started participating in a local book club with other dementia patients and their caregivers, he saw a marked improvement in his overall health. His blood pressure levels were better regulated, and he seemed happier and more engaged. Just like Mr. Brown, your loved one could also reap these benefits.

Being socially active is about more than just the physical aspect, though. It's also a buffer against mental health conditions that often accompany dementia, like depression and anxiety. Take Mrs. White, for example. She was a woman who loved painting. After her Alzheimer's diagnosis, her family encouraged her to join an art class for seniors with similar conditions. Painting with others not only allowed her to express herself artistically but also brought joy and meaning to her life. Her sleep improved, and she was less anxious, more present, and more content.

Social interaction also helps seniors maintain their independence. Imagine your loved one in a community where they can express their feelings freely, surrounded by friends and caregivers who understand their condition. This support system can bolster their self-confidence, providing them with a renewed sense of purpose.

Remember, communication isn't always verbal. It could be through shared activities. Think about your loved one's hobbies and interests. Could they paint, like Mrs. White? Or enjoy music, dance, or even simple household tasks?

Creative Approaches to Engaging with People with Dementia

"Every person's life is like a tapestry, woven with many threads, each of which brings its own hue and texture to the whole." We all carry within us a unique blend of memories, experiences, and passions that shape who we are. Yet, as we age, some of these threads may begin to fray or fade. This is particularly true for those living with dementia, a condition that affects millions of people worldwide. But as someone who has walked this path with a loved one, I want to share with you that while dementia may change the nature of the threads, it does not mean the tapestry is complete.

From my journey and extensive research, I've gathered a wealth of knowledge about creative and effective ways to engage with people living with dementia. These strategies aim to honor the rich tapestry that makes up each person's life, cherishing their dignity and individuality and, importantly, helping to keep them engaged and active in ways that are both meaningful and enjoyable.

Let's start with outdoor activities. There's something profoundly healing about nature. It can awaken our senses, uplift our spirits, and reconnect us with the world in a way that feels grounding and soothing. A simple walk in the park or courtyard can be transformed into an enriching experience by paying attention to the surroundings - the color of flowers, the smell of fresh grass, and the rustling of leaves in the wind. For my father, who was an avid birdwatcher, pointing out different birds and their songs was a joyful activity that rekindled happy memories. If mobility is an issue, you could set up a comfortable spot in the yard where you and your loved one can sit and enjoy the fresh air and natural sights.

Indoor activities can be just as fulfilling. Music, for instance, has a powerful way of reaching parts of our brain that other forms of communication cannot. Playing their favorite songs from the past can stir emotions and memories. My mother, for instance, could remember and hum along to the melodies of songs she used to dance to in her youth, even when she struggled to recall other aspects of her past. Similarly, sorting and matching up nuts and bolts or tightening screws into pieces of wood can provide a sense of accomplishment and tap into their former interests or professions. For my father, who was a mechanic, this simple task brought immense joy and a sense of purpose.

Personal activities can play a crucial role too. Simple self-care tasks like brushing their teeth or selecting an outfit can provide a sense of control and normalcy. You might be surprised how much pride and satisfaction a person with dementia can derive from independently accomplishing these small, everyday tasks.

In the kitchen, we can stimulate the senses and evoke memories. The smell of a favorite meal cooking or the texture of dough can spark joy and recollections. Baking cookies with my grandmother, for instance, was an activity she thoroughly enjoyed. It gave her a sense of purpose and allowed us to bond over shared experiences.

Lastly, family traditions can be a powerful way of connecting with your loved one. These can range from holiday rituals to weekly family dinners. My family always gathered around the table on Sunday evenings for a meal. Even as my father's memory faded, this tradition remained a source of comfort and familiarity for him.

Practical Tips for Improving Communication and Connection

Remember the classic story of the Tower of Babel? Where language, once a common thread that bound humanity, suddenly became a source of confusion and discord? Living with a loved one suffering from dementia can sometimes feel like living in the aftermath of the Tower of Babel, where communication, once straightforward and effortless, becomes mired in misunderstanding and frustration. But unlike in the story, where humanity had to scatter and adapt to their new linguistic isolation, you and your loved one can find ways to bridge the communication gap that dementia tends to create.

Dementia diseases often bring a slew of changes in communication skills. It's as if the person you've known and loved for years is suddenly speaking a different language; a language fraught with forgotten words, lost trains of thought, and confusion over meanings. It is understandable to yearn for the days when conversations flowed effortlessly, and words were not such elusive entities.

You might notice your loved one having trouble finding the right word or losing their train of thought mid-sentence. They may struggle to comprehend what certain words mean or find it challenging to focus during prolonged conversations. In certain situations, individuals with dementia may struggle to remember the steps involved in routine activities, such as cooking a meal, managing finances, or dressing themselves.

You may also notice that they're more easily distracted by background noises, such as the radio, TV, or other conversations.

This increased sensitivity can often lead to frustration when communication doesn't flow as smoothly as it used to.

In some cases, dementia can cause people to revert to their first language, especially if English was learned as a second language. This can add another layer of complexity to your communication efforts, but don't lose heart. With understanding and a few practical strategies, you can make communication easier for both you and your loved one.

Firstly, recognize that these changes in communication skills are a result of the disease and not a reflection of your loved one's desire or ability to communicate with you.

When you talk to them, make eye contact, and call them by their name. This can help ground them in the moment and foster a more meaningful connection.

Your tone of voice, facial expressions, and body language can also significantly impact how your messages are received. Try to maintain a calm, positive demeanor, even when you feel frustrated or impatient.

Encourage two-way conversations for as long as possible. Even if it's challenging to understand your loved one's thoughts, your willingness to listen and engage can provide them with a sense of normalcy and emotional support.

In addition to speaking, consider using other forms of communication, such as gentle touch or visual aids. If you find that communication is causing undue stress or agitation, distraction can be a useful tool. For instance, you could redirect their attention to a favorite song or a photo album.

To better communicate with a person who has dementia, you'll need to simplify your language and be direct, specific, and positive in your interactions.

For example, instead of saying, "Don't do this," say, "Please do this." Offer simple, step-by-step instructions, and repeat them as necessary, allowing ample time for a response. Avoid "baby talk," but try to articulate your words clearly and slowly to ensure understanding.

Phrase your questions to require a 'yes' or 'no' response, such as, "Are you tired?" instead of "How do you feel?" Limit choices to avoid overwhelming them. For example, instead of asking, "What would you like for dinner?" ask, "Would you like a hamburger or chicken for dinner?"

If you feel frustrated, it's important to take a timeout for yourself. Remember, caregiving is a marathon, not a sprint.

Non-Verbal Communication and Dementia

I still remember when I was a young girl, my grandfather, a proud and reserved man, would sit quietly in his favorite armchair, a book always in his hands. Yet, it was not his words that told us how he felt; it was the subtle raising of his eyebrows, the firmness of his grip on the book, and the slight nod of his head. His silence spoke volumes; as a child, I learned to listen, understand, and decipher his non-verbal cues. Years later, when dementia took away his ability to communicate with words, these memories guided me as I navigated the new language he spoke — a language of silence, gestures, and emotions.

Communicating with a loved one with dementia can be a deeply challenging and emotionally intense experience. One of the greatest hurdles you may face is the progressive loss of verbal communication abilities. However, as my experience with my grandfather taught me, when words fail, other forms of communication come into play. This is the world of non-verbal communication.

Non-verbal communication, as the name suggests, is a form of interaction that doesn't rely on spoken or written words.

Instead, it revolves around things like facial expressions, body language, and physical gestures. We all use non-verbal communication to some extent in our everyday lives. You may use it when you smile at a neighbor, cross your arms in a meeting, or hug a friend in need. In the context of dementia, it becomes even more crucial as it might become the primary way for your loved one to express themselves.

Think of it as a silent conversation. When verbal abilities decline, your loved one may start to use gestures or facial expressions to communicate their feelings or needs. They might not tell you that they're sad, but their eyes might well up with tears. They might not say they're confused, but their furrowed brows could be trying to communicate just that. As a caregiver, understanding and responding to these silent signals can make all the difference.

Let me share some practical strategies to enhance your non-verbal communication skills while interacting with your loved one who has dementia. These tips are not one-size-fits-all solutions, but they can offer a starting point to help you navigate this challenging journey.

One of the most comforting forms of non-verbal communication is physical contact. It's a universal language that can convey love, reassurance, and companionship. A gentle touch on the arm, a warm hand on their shoulder, or holding their hand can communicate your presence and care. It's a tangible way to say, "I'm here for you." However, always be mindful of their comfort and personal boundaries.

While physical proximity can be comforting, too much closeness can sometimes feel intrusive or intimidating. To avoid this, try to maintain a respectful distance when communicating. Instead of standing over them, sit or stand at their eye level. This can help foster a sense of equality and mutual respect.

Remember, just as you observe their non-verbal cues, they also read yours. Your body language, facial expressions, and even the tone of your voice can convey a multitude of messages. It's essential to ensure that your non-verbal signals align with your spoken words. For instance, if you're reminiscing about a joyful memory, let your face reflect that joy with a warm smile.

A key part of non-verbal communication is being observant and responsive to the other person's cues. If they seem uncomfortable or disinterested, adjust your approach. If they seem relaxed and engaged, continue in that vein. Remember, this is a two-way street, and your loved one may be trying to communicate their feelings and needs through their body language.

Alzheimer's Caregiving: Changes in Communication Skills

In 2003, a story captured the hearts of many when an elderly couple's love stood the test of time and adversity. Bob DeMarco dedicated his life to caring for his mother, Dotty, who had Alzheimer's. With unwavering patience, he navigated the challenging landscape of her fading memory and changing personality. His experience, chronicled in their shared journey through dementia, holds lessons for us all. It reminds us that when words fail, when memories fade, our actions and our patience can speak volumes.

I understand that communicating with a loved one who has Alzheimer's can be an incredibly personal and challenging experience. Communication serves as the foundation of our relationships, allowing us to express our thoughts, feelings, needs, and desires, and fostering connection. However, Alzheimer's disease can pose significant challenges to communication, leading to frustration and misunderstandings.

One of the primary hurdles you might face is changes in your loved one's communication abilities. They may struggle to find the right words, lose their train of thought mid-conversation, or have difficulty understanding what words mean. They might also have a hard time paying attention during longer conversations, forgetting the steps in common activities, or become sensitive to background noises. Some individuals may also revert to their first language if English was learned as a second language. Remember, these changes are a result of the disease and not a reflection of your loved one's desire to communicate with you.

So, how do you make communication easier with your loved one with Alzheimer's? It starts with making eye contact and calling them by their name. Engaging in this simple act of attentiveness can assist individuals with Alzheimer's in focusing and feeling acknowledged. Be mindful of your tone of voice, the volume at which you speak, your facial expressions, and your body language. These non-verbal cues can significantly impact communication and help create a more positive and understanding interaction. These cues often communicate more than our words do.

Encourage a two-way conversation for as long as possible. Resist the urge to finish their sentences or rush them. Patience here is key. Remember, their thought process might take a little longer now, and that's okay.

You can also use other methods of communication aside from speaking. Gentle touching, like holding their hand, can be comforting and reassuring. If communication becomes particularly challenging, try distraction. A change in activity or environment can help reset their mood.

Encouraging your loved one to communicate with you can be nurtured in a warm, loving, and understanding manner. Let them feel heard, even if they are hard to understand. Allow them to make decisions and stay involved in day-to-day activities as much as possible. This can help maintain their sense of independence and dignity.

When your loved one has an angry outburst, be patient. It's the illness talking, not them. They may be struggling with feelings they can't express or understand.

When speaking with a person who has Alzheimer's, be direct, specific, and positive. Offer simple, step-by-step instructions and repeat them if necessary. Try not to talk about the person as if they aren't there or resort to using "baby talk."

Always acknowledge their efforts and express gratitude. Instead of saying, "Don't do this," say, "Please do this," or replace "You've made a mistake" with "Let's try this way." Positivity can help reinforce their self-esteem and reduce frustration.

If your loved one is aware of their memory loss, they may want to talk about the changes they're noticing. Be sensitive and patient, listen to them, and try not to correct them whenever they forget or say something odd. Help them find words to express their thoughts and feelings, but don't rush to fill in the blanks too quickly.

Summary Box

Chapter 5: Connecting Through the Fog delved into the pivotal role of social and emotional connections for people with dementia. As humans, we are inherently social beings. Our relationships, our connections, and our interactions with others give life its color and flavor. For those grappling with dementia, these connections become even more crucial.

The isolation and confusion that dementia often brings can be disorienting, even frightening. It's like waking up to a dense fog where familiar paths have vanished, and every step feels uncertain. But it's through the warm hand of connection that this fog can be pierced. It's the power of connection that can usher in rays of recognition, comfort, and calm.

One of the key aspects we explored in this chapter is the importance of social interaction for those with Alzheimer's and other forms of dementia. Regular social interaction can slow the progression of the disease and improve the quality of life. It's not just about staving off loneliness; it's about preserving their sense of self, their identity.

As you navigate this journey with your loved one, I shared some creative approaches to engaging with people with dementia. The disease might have changed how they interact with the world. Still, it doesn't diminish their capacity to experience joy, love, and fulfillment.

From simple activities like looking through old photo albums or listening to their favorite music to more elaborate ones like art therapy or pet therapy, there are myriad ways to connect with your loved one. These activities can bring back cherished memories, stimulate their senses, and even spark moments of clarity and cognizance.

Improving communication and connection with your loved one is an ongoing process. It's about learning, adapting, and improvising. In this chapter, I shared practical tips to enhance your communication skills.

We delved into the significance of non-verbal communication in dementia care. When words become elusive, body language, facial expressions, and tone of voice often become the primary means of expression for those with dementia. Learning to understand and respond to these non-verbal cues can help you connect with your loved one in a deeper, more meaningful way.

The chapter also covered changes in communication skills for caregiving. From understanding these changes to adapting your communication style, these insights will help you navigate the winding paths of dementia communication.

As we journeyed through this chapter, I hope you found strategies and insights that illuminated your path. May these words serve as a beacon, guiding you as you reach out to your loved one, connecting through the fog of dementia.

Segue:

As we close the chapter on 'Connecting Through the Fog,' let's pause for a moment and reflect on the journey we've taken so far. We've explored the intricacies of dementia care, the labyrinth of emotions, challenges, and rewards it presents. We've delved into the profound role of social and emotional connections for those living with dementia and how these connections, these lifelines, can light their path even when the fog of confusion sets in.

We've discussed how important social interactions are, not just for the comfort and companionship they provide but also for preserving their sense of self and identity. We've shared creative ways to engage and connect with your loved ones, to kindle sparks of recognition, joy, and fulfillment amidst the haze of dementia.

We've delved into the subtleties of non-verbal communication, the silent language of facial expressions, body language, and tone of voice that often become the primary means of expression for your loved ones. And we've navigated the shifting landscape of communication skills in caregiving, understanding the changes and learning to adapt and improvise.

Every insight, every tip, and every strategy we've shared is a steppingstone, a beacon to guide you as you journey through the labyrinth of dementia care. Each one is a testament to your resilience, your compassion, and your unwavering commitment to your loved ones.

But remember, dear reader, while these strategies and insights can illuminate your path, it's your love, your patience, and your empathy that truly make the difference. It's in the gentle squeeze of your hand, the patient repetition of a familiar story, the soft lullaby that eases them into sleep - these are the moments that pierce through the fog, that reach out to your loved one in their silent world.

As we transition into the next chapter, we're going to embrace a new perspective, a new lens through which to view this journey. We've walked through the fog, hand in hand with our loved ones. We've navigated the twists and turns, the highs and lows. Now, it's time to step back, to look at the journey in its entirety.

In the next chapter, 'Embracing the Journey,' we will explore how to hold this journey with grace and resilience. We'll delve into the transformative power of acceptance, of finding peace amidst the storm. We'll look at how to turn challenges into opportunities for growth, deepening our connections, and discovering strengths we never knew we had.

So, take a deep breath, dear reader. Take a moment to recognize and appreciate the progress you have made on this journey. And when you're ready, join me on this next leg of our journey as we learn to embrace the twists and turns, the ups and downs, and the beautiful chaos that is the maze of dementia care.

Chapter 6:
Embracing the Journey

Please note that information about the resources mentioned in this chapter can be found on the Resource page at the end of the book.

"Physical strength is measured by what we can carry; spiritual by what we can bear." — Unknown

Positive Aspects of Dementia Caregiving and Experiences

As I sat down to write this section of the book, I couldn't help but remember a quote that resonated with me throughout my journey as a caregiver: "In the midst of difficulty lies opportunity." —Albert Einstein. Indeed, caregiving for someone with dementia can be a profoundly challenging experience. However, it is equally important to acknowledge and recognize the positive aspects that can emerge from this journey.

I remember when I first began taking care of my parents, both of whom suffered from dementia, I was overwhelmed by the stress and uncertainty of the situation. However, over time, I learned that there were silver linings in this journey. I discovered a deeper sense of purpose and a profound appreciation for the human spirit.

One of the most rewarding aspects of dementia caregiving is indeed the chance to shift our focus from the disease itself to the person living with it. This shift in perspective allows us to see the individual's strengths and capabilities rather than just their limitations. For instance, during my mother's battle with dementia, I was amazed by her ability to remember the lyrics of her favorite songs, even when she couldn't recall my name. By focusing on these small victories, I was able to find joy and meaning in our journey together.

Working together as a team with other family members, friends, and healthcare professionals is another positive aspect of dementia caregiving. This collaboration not only lightens the load for the primary caregiver but also fosters a sense of community and support. I remember the countless times my siblings and I would come together to share stories, laughter, and tears as we navigated our way through the challenges of caring for our parents.

The COVID-19 pandemic presented unprecedented challenges for dementia caregivers, but it also highlighted the resilience and adaptability of caregivers and their loved ones.

During the pandemic, respecting the personhood of those living with dementia became even more crucial as we were forced to adapt to new routines and ways of connecting.

By tapping into our loved ones' virtues and values, we were able to maintain a sense of continuity and familiarity. For example, my good friend had always been a devout Christian, so we made a point to involve him in virtual church services during the lockdown. This helped him feel connected to his faith and provided a sense of stability during a chaotic time.

The pandemic also taught us the importance of seeking and receiving support from our network of friends, family, and healthcare professionals. Connecting with others who were going through similar experiences, either in person or through online forums, provided much-needed emotional support and encouragement.

Additionally, the pandemic underscored the necessity of prioritizing self-care for caregivers. As the saying goes, "You can't pour from an empty cup." Taking time for ourselves, whether it be through exercise, meditation, or hobbies, allowed us to recharge our batteries and be more effective caregivers.

Being protective and proactive in our approach to dementia care during the pandemic meant making practical changes to ensure the safety and well-being of our loved ones. This included learning about and implementing infection control measures, modifying living spaces, and staying informed about the latest recommendations from healthcare professionals.

As we emerge from the pandemic, we can reflect on the lessons learned and use them to strengthen our commitment to the person living with dementia. This includes continuing to focus on their needs and well-being while also looking after our own needs as caregivers.

Mind-Body-Spirit Approaches to Dementia Care

Mindfulness is a state of mind in which you purposefully direct your attention to the present moment without passing judgment on your thoughts or experiences. It might sound simple, but our minds often race ahead to future tasks or linger in the past, making it difficult to stay present. Mindfulness techniques, such as focusing on your breath or the sensations in your body, can be helpful in anchoring you to the present moment.

Now, let's discuss how mindfulness can help you in your caregiving journey:

1. Reducing stress and anxiety in both you and the person you're caring for.

When you practice mindfulness, it can help you feel calmer and more at ease. This state of mind has been linked to improved mental and physical health. As you remain calm, your loved one with dementia will likely sense your calmness and feel more relaxed as well. Your ability to manage situations thoughtfully, rather than reacting impulsively, can make a significant difference in your caregiving experience.

2. Increasing concentration and reducing the likelihood of making mistakes.

As caregivers, we often find ourselves multitasking. However, constantly juggling tasks can be mentally exhausting and increases the likelihood of making mistakes. Mindfulness helps you focus on one task at a time, reducing mental fatigue and the chance of errors. By being fully present in each task, you can complete it more efficiently and accurately.

3. Supporting better self-care.

Caregivers often neglect their own well-being, but mindfulness can help change that. By being more aware of your present experience, you can recognize when you're tired or emotionally drained and take the necessary steps to care for yourself. It also allows you to break the cycle of negative thoughts and focus on what's happening in the present moment.

- Integrating mindfulness into your daily routine doesn't need to be complicated. Here are a few straightforward ways to practice mindfulness throughout your day:

- Mindful breathing: Dedicating a few moments to focus on your breath. Notice the feeling of the air entering and leaving your body, the rise and fall of your chest or abdomen, or any other physical sensations associated with your breath. When you notice your mind wandering, gently and non-judgmentally bring your focus back to your breath. This practice helps foster mindfulness, bringing you into the present moment and promoting a sense of calm and clarity.

- Mindful eating: Pay close attention to the flavors, textures, and sensations of each bite when you have a meal or snack. Chew slowly and savor the experience.

- Mindful pauses: Take short breaks during the day to pause and tune into your present moment. Notice the sensations in your body, the sounds around you, and the thoughts passing through your mind.

- Mindful walking: While walking, bring your attention to the physical sensations of each step. Feel the ground beneath your feet, the movement of your body, and the sights and sounds of your surroundings.

- Mindful gratitude: Practice gratitude by intentionally acknowledging and appreciating the things you are grateful for in your life. It could be as simple as expressing gratitude for a beautiful sunrise or a kind gesture from a loved one.

- Mindful self-compassion: It is important to cultivate self-kindness and compassion in your daily life. Treat yourself with the same care, compassion, and understanding that you would extend to a close friend or loved one.

- Remember, mindfulness is about being fully present in the moment, without judgment. By incorporating these simple practices into your daily routine, you can improve your sense of awareness, peace, and well-being.

- Take three deep breaths several times a day, focusing on the sensation of the breath in your body.

- When doing chores, pay full attention to the task at hand. For example, if you're washing dishes, focus on the sensation of the soapy water on your skin.

- When you hear a siren or other loud noise, stop, and listen to the sound, noting its quality, volume, and the silence that follows.

- While brushing your teeth, concentrate on the sensation in your arm as you hold the brush or the bristles on your teeth, gums, and tongue.

Mindfulness Meditation

To begin practicing mindfulness meditation, find a comfortable position with your eyes closed or softly focused on a point in front of you. Set an intention for your practice, such as cultivating patience or bettering your health. Take three full breaths and then return to a natural breath. Focus your attention on your breath, labeling it "in, out, in, out" or "rising, falling." When you feel your attention is steady, let go of these "subtitles" and experience your breath just as it is, being aware that you are aware.

As you practice, it's natural for your mind to wander. When you notice you're no longer paying attention to your breath, gently bring your focus back. This act of catching yourself and returning to the present moment is the essence of the practice. If a difficult emotion arises, try using the RAIN technique to mindfully manage it:

1. *Recognize* - Acknowledge what you are feeling and gently label it non-judgmentally.

2. *Allowing (Acceptance)* - Be willing to be present with your experience, no matter how unpleasant.

3. *Investigate* - Witness the emotion with kindness and from an unbiased perspective.

4. *Non-Identification* - Recognize that you are not this emotion; it is just a temporary event.

Remember, mindfulness meditation is a practice, not a performance. It's normal to get distracted, but the key is to start over with a gentle and kind attitude towards yourself. Try incorporating informal awareness breaks into your day, like taking a deep breath or paying attention to the sensation of your hands on the steering wheel. Even a few seconds of mindfulness can help interrupt the stress response and bring more peace and health into your life.

Concentrative Meditation

(Can also be done with the patient)

My journey as a caregiver for my parents, who had dementia, taught me many valuable lessons, and one of them was the importance of self-care. One of the tools that helped me tremendously was concentrative meditation. I found that not only did it provide me with a sense of calm and focus, but it also allowed me to share moments of peace and connection with my loved ones as they battled dementia. I would like to share this with you so that you, too, can find solace in the midst of the challenges you face as a caregiver.

Concentrative meditation is a practice that aims to help you settle your mind and still your body by focusing on a single thought or object. Just as a laser-like focus can empower you to achieve your goals and dreams, concentrative meditation can help you develop mental clarity and resilience in the face of adversity.

There are four types of concentrative meditation, and I encourage you to explore each one to find what resonates most with you and your loved one with dementia.

1. *Meditating on your breath:* This type of meditation involves focusing on your inhalation and exhalation. As you pay attention to your breath, you become more aware of your connection to life and the world around you. This practice can be especially beneficial when you're feeling overwhelmed, as it helps to calm your mind and body. You can also share this

meditation with your loved one, guiding them to focus on their breath as well.

2. *Focusing on a sound:* In this type of meditation, you concentrate on a sound, such as a mantra, a word, or even a song. Instead of chanting the sound aloud, you mentally recall it, imagining your mind saying or hearing the sound. This practice can help you break free from the distractions and restlessness that often accompany caregiving.

3. *Meditating on a form of your choice:* To meditate on a form, you visualize a specific object or image, like a peaceful landscape or a religious icon. As you focus on the form, you might find that your mental image fades away. This is normal. Simply refresh your visualization by opening your eyes, looking at the form again, and closing your eyes or taking a deep breath. The goal is to maintain the form in your mental eye for as long as possible.

4. *Meditating on the formless:* This type of meditation is more advanced and involves achieving a state of thoughtlessness. You don't visualize anything; instead, you sit in a state of natural balance, exertion, and relaxation. It may take more practice than the other forms of meditation, but it can lead to a profound sense of bliss and expanded consciousness.

As a caregiver, you might feel isolated and overwhelmed at times. Incorporating concentrative meditation into your daily routine can offer you a much-needed moment of peace and clarity. I found that sharing these moments with my loved ones, even as they struggled with dementia, brought us closer and helped us find meaning and joy in our journey together. Give it a try and remember that you are not alone.

Positive Affirmations

When I first started caring for my parents, I often overlooked my well-being, which took a toll on my mental and emotional health. I learned that to effectively care for my loved one, I needed to take care of myself as well. Through the practice of positive affirmations, I was able to shift my focus away from negative emotions and direct it toward my strengths and the small joys in life.

Positive affirmations are simple statements that help you focus on the good things in your life and yourself. Repeating these affirmations can boost your confidence, inspire, and encourage you, decrease feelings of anxiety, and even influence your subconscious mind to access new beliefs.

Here are some of the affirmations that I found helpful during my time as a caregiver:

- I learn every day from the mistakes I make

- My life is full of joy, peace, and love

- I am valuable and important

- I invite abundance and happiness into my life

- My body is healthy, happy, and radiant

- I am a caring and compassionate caregiver

- My future is full of happiness and laughter

- I am grateful for everything I have

- I will allow myself to change and evolve

- My life is full of learning and growth

- I am courageous and relentless

- I deserve to rest and recharge

- My smile radiates positivity

- My care and love have healing powers

- I will not stress about the future

- I find joy in caring for my elderly loved one

- I will find happiness in the care and service

- My love is pure and unconditional

- I see so many positives in caregiving

In addition to helping me maintain my own well-being, positive affirmations also played a significant role in strengthening the relationship between my parents and me. By practicing these affirmations, I was able to respond to their needs in a more positive and compassionate manner, which ultimately improved our bond.

Even in relationships where there is resistance to change or denial of the challenges faced, positive affirmations can still help. By making a conscious effort to focus on the positive aspects and remaining calm in the face of adversity, you can bring about a slow but steady improvement in your relationship with your loved one.

Positive affirmations can also have a ripple effect on those around you. When you respond to others with kindness and understanding, you can influence them to adopt a more positive outlook as well. As a caregiver, this can be particularly powerful in fostering a strong and supportive bond with your loved one.

Some encouraging affirmations to help strengthen your relationship include:

- I am blessed to have this relationship in my life

- The more love I give, the more love I will receive in this relationship

- I am eternally grateful for your friendship

- I treat my relationship with the care and respect it deserves

- My heart is always overflowing with gratitude for our special bond

- I feel free to be myself in our relationship

- We respect and appreciate our relationship

- I love the healthy boundaries in our relationship

- I admire and respect the care and love you show me

- We understand and appreciate all the effort that is put into this relationship

- I deserve all the love, respect, and care I get in this relationship

- I am mindful of the time and attention I get

Physical Meditation

Yoga for Dementia Caregivers

As a caregiver for my loved ones with dementia, I have experienced firsthand the challenges and stresses that come with this role. It's crucial for caregivers like us to find ways to manage our stress, maintain our mental and physical well-being, and preserve our capacity to care for our loved ones. One effective way to do this is through regular yoga practice, which can provide immense benefits for the body and spirit.

In my journey as a caregiver, I've found that yoga has been a great way to soothe my heart, mind, and body. Giving care, whether it's to a baby, a sick partner, an aging parent, or as part of a career, is a sacred act. We offer our time, presence, and energy to someone else, and this powerful gift can take a toll on us, especially when it means watching someone we care about suffer.

To care well, we need to access the softness in our hearts that allows us to feel compassion and empathy. We also need firm boundaries to protect this softness. When we don't protect our capacity to care, we can lose that softness altogether, leading to compassion fatigue. This can be dangerous, particularly when someone is relying on us.

Taking care of our physical bodies is crucial in this journey. I've noticed that, as caregivers, we often experience tightness in the upper back region, as well as the hips, especially when caring for someone who is suffering. Stress and anxiety can cause the belly to contract, pulling the legs in towards the body. Releasing the front of the hips can help release this stress.

A regular yoga practice nourishes the body and spirit, and even a little bit can make a huge difference. Here are some postures I've found particularly helpful in my own experience as a caregiver:

1. *Self-Love Meditation:* In a comfortable seated position or lying down, place one hand over your heart and the other hand over the first hand. Breathe deeply, focusing on yourself and

your own well-being. Remain in this meditation for 3–10 minutes.

2. *Supported Fish:* This restorative posture opens the front of the heart and chest, as well as the belly. Lay back onto a bolster, cushion, or pillows allowing your arms to open to the sides and your chest to gently open. Breathe deeply and remain in this posture for 2–20 minutes.

3. *Supine Twist:* This twist helps release tension in the shoulders, spine, hips, and digestive system. Lay on your right side with your knees up in line with your hips, then roll your left arm open to the left, allowing your shoulder to come to the floor. Stay for 5–10 breaths and switch sides.

4. *Gentle Core:* Engage your abdominal muscles to help support your back and provide a sense of strength and protection. Lay on your back with your knees bent and feet on the floor, and gently engage your pelvic floor muscles and lower belly as you exhale. Optionally, lift your upper back off the ground and alternate lifting your feet off the floor.

5. *Cat/Cow:* This movement helps stretch the spine and can be done on all fours or seated. Inhale deeply as you arch your back, and exhale fully as you round your back. Repeat 5–10 times.

6. *Standing Forward Bend:* This pose releases back and neck tension, as well as stretching the back and hamstrings. Stand with your feet hip-distance apart and fold over your legs, allowing your neck to relax completely. Stay for 5–20 breaths.

7. *Twisted High Lunge:* This pose helps release the psoas muscle, which is related to stress, and provides a gentle massage for the internal organs.

Tai Chi for Dementia Caregivers

I recall a memorable moment when my nephew, a master of martial arts, told me about a legendary martial arts master who lived in a small village in China. His name was lost to history, but his legacy lived on in his teachings. He was old, older than anyone else in the village, yet he moved with the grace and agility of a young man. Every morning, as the sun rose, he would perform a series of flowing movements in the village square. Villagers, young and old, would gather to watch him, mesmerized by the elegance and tranquility he exuded. He explained that his secret was an ancient martial art known as Tai Chi, a practice he said was like "medication in motion."

In this section, I want to share with you the benefits of Tai Chi, can effectively help in maintaining strength, flexibility, and balance. Engaging in this activity can be beneficial not only as a caregiver but also for the entirety of your life. It has the potential to foster resilience, helping you navigate the challenges that come with dementia care.

Imagine standing amidst the flowering trees in a peaceful park, holding a Tai Chi pose as the sun rises. The serenity and connection to nature are part of the whole experience. Tai Chi, often described as "meditation in motion," originated in China as a martial art. However, it has evolved and is now recognized for its potential in treating or preventing many health problems.

The beauty of Tai Chi lies in its low-impact, slow-motion exercise. It's a series of motions named for animal actions like "white crane spreads its wings" or martial arts moves such as "box both ears." Throughout the movements, you breathe deeply and naturally, focusing your attention on your bodily sensations. The movements are typically circular and never forced, with muscles relaxed rather than tensed, and joints not fully extended or bent. It's an exercise form that can be easily adapted for anyone, from the fittest among us to those confined to wheelchairs or recovering from surgery.

Tai Chi is more than just an exercise; it is a practice that is part of a broader philosophy. Though you don't need to delve deep into Chinese philosophy to enjoy the benefits of Tai Chi, understanding the underlying concepts can enrich the experience:

Qi is believed to be an energy force that flows through the body. Tai Chi, a martial art and form of exercise, is said to unblock and encourage the proper flow of Qi. Additionally, Yin and Yang are opposing elements that are believed to make up the universe, and maintaining harmony between them is considered important. Tai Chi is thought to promote this balance by incorporating gentle and flowing movements that help cultivate harmony and equilibrium in both the body and mind

Your Tai Chi journey could start with a simple warm-up, including easy motions like shoulder circles, turning the head from side to side, or rocking back and forth. These movements help loosen your muscles and joints and focus on your breath and body. Once you're warmed up, you will move on to the practice of Tai Chi forms. These forms are sets of movements — short forms may include a dozen or fewer movements, and long forms may include hundreds.

Qigong, which can be translated as "breath work" or "energy work," often involves a few minutes of gentle breathing exercises combined with movement. The purpose of Qigong is to promote relaxation of the mind and mobilize the body's energy.

By incorporating intentional breathing techniques and gentle movements, Qigong aims to cultivate a sense of calm, enhance mental focus, and harmonize the body's energy flow. It is considered a holistic practice that encompasses physical, mental, and energetic aspects of well-being.

Starting your Tai Chi journey is simple. You don't need any fancy equipment, and it's easy to practice at home or in a local class. One piece of advice I'd like to share is not to be intimidated by the language. Different branches of Tai Chi, such as Yang, Wu, and Cheng, are named after the individuals who developed specific sets of movements called forms within those styles. However, it is important to note that the name of the style is not as significant as finding an approach that aligns with your interests and needs.

Mental Imagery

In my younger days, my mother used to tell me a story about a brave knight who would journey far and wide to protect his kingdom. Despite the many battles he fought, the countless hours he spent training, and the sleepless nights spent on patrol, he was never too weary to care for his people. Now, as I look back, I realize that the story was not just about bravery or duty. It was about caregiving, about the strength it takes to be there for others, and about the power of self-care. As a caregiver to my loved ones who suffered from dementia, I understand the significance of those lessons more than ever.

Let's now delve into some strategies that helped me during my journey and might assist you on yours. I call this 'Imagery for Caregivers.' This practice is designed specifically for anyone who is or has been a caregiver. While the rewards of caring for a friend or loved one with an illness can be very meaningful, it often requires a remarkable effort.

Imagine yourself seated comfortably or perhaps lying down on your back on the floor or a bed. Align your head, neck, and shoulders in a manner that feels supported. Now, start focusing on your breathing. There's no need to force it, simply inhale a refreshing breath and exhale fully. In this moment, you're not needed by anyone, anywhere, for anything. This is a time for you to release and receive.

Thoughts or feelings might surface, trying to compete for your attention. But there's no need to engage, just focus on your breath and let any thoughts or emotions pass through like bubbles floating to the surface and releasing.

As you continue to breathe, inhale peace and calm, and exhale any tension or discomfort you may be holding. With each breath, release any weariness and receive replenishment. Feel your muscles soften, and your joints loosen, creating capacity for each cleansing and rejuvenating breath.

Remember my mother's story about the brave knight? Now it's time for you to journey to a place where you have no worries or responsibilities. A place free of concern or schedules. It might be a place you've visited or dreamed of visiting. It could be your current home or even the familiar settings of your childhood.

You're on this journey, and as you draw nearer to this carefree destination, let your senses take it in. Maybe you're at a beach, in a fresh meadow, or in your favorite room of your home. Take in the colors, the aromas, the sounds, the light. Feel the sensations, perhaps a breeze or the popping crackle of a fire, or maybe a mountain trail or sandy beach beneath your feet. In this moment, you are safe, comfortable, and free.

Picture a time when you provided care for a loved one or friend. Connect with the sense of care and love you have for that person. What do you notice about your experience of providing care? Allow the deep care and respect that direct your actions to be present. If emotions arise, there's no need to engage; let them simply pass through you.

As you recall your caregiving, notice your voice, your skill, and maybe even your sense of humor. You are transmitting caring, comforting, healing attention, and energy toward this person. Note where this energy comes from. Is it from within you? Is there anything you need to do to keep replenishing this energy, this intent, this ability?

Apps for Meditation

In the past, I've often found myself grappling with the overwhelming stress of caring for my loved ones afflicted with dementia. I remember one evening after a particularly challenging day, I sat down, feeling the weight of the world on my shoulders. It was then that I discovered the magic of meditation, a practice that not only provided me solace but became a cornerstone of my caregiving journey.

Sharing this personal experience with you, I understand that your caregiving journey is likely as demanding and stressful as mine was, if not more. The physical and mental toll on you is immense, leaving you drained and often dispirited. But I want to assure you that there is a simple, effective tool that can significantly improve your well-being: meditation.

Meditation is a practice that is easily accessible to everyone. You don't need any special equipment or expensive classes. All you need is a quiet spot where you can sit, breathe, and focus your attention on a way that helps your body and mind relax. Guided meditations are a wonderful starting point, as you can follow the calming voice prompts that help you navigate the process.

Don't worry if your thoughts wander while you're meditating; that happens to everyone. The key is simply to do it without worrying about whether you're doing it "right" or "wrong." With time, you'll find your rhythm and your unique way of meditating that resonates with you.

The benefits of meditation are many, some of which I've personally experienced. Regular meditation can help regulate your emotions, reduce the physical effects of stress, and even boost your immune system. It has helped me improve my sleep, reduce feelings of depression, and lower my blood pressure.

In today's technologically advanced world, there are numerous apps available that make meditation easy and convenient. I've found these four apps to be especially beneficial and user-friendly for caregivers like you and me:

1. *Insight Timer:* This is one of the most popular free meditation apps. With nearly 7,000 free guided meditations from thousands of teachers, you're spoilt for choice. You can choose

meditations based on topic or by length of time, which can be as short as 0 - 5 minutes. The app also has a community aspect, letting you see how many people are meditating right now and even inviting friends to join.

2. *Smiling Mind:* Hailing from Australia, Smiling Mind is a not-for-profit organization dedicated to making mindfulness meditation accessible to everyone. Their meditations, all of which are free, range in focus and length, with some being just one minute long – perfect for fitting into even the busiest days.

3. *Sanvello:* This app is a toolset to reduce and manage stress, anxiety, and depression, providing techniques based on cognitive behavioral therapy and mindfulness. It helps you cope with difficult situations and emotions, and even allows you to track your thoughts, mood, health, and goals.

4. *Headspace:* Perfect for beginners, Headspace eases you into meditation with a helpful Basics course. It's a great app for those wanting more tips on how to get started with meditation.

Remember, meditation isn't about perfection; it's about practice. Every small effort you put into it counts. I encourage you to explore these apps, find the ones that resonate with you, and make meditation a part of your daily routine. This simple practice could be the key to finding the resilience, peace, and strength you need in your caregiving journey.

Spirituality and Faith in Dementia Care

In the hushed stillness of the predawn hours, as the world slumbered and the stars held sway over the sky, I would often find myself sitting by my father's bedside, holding his frail hand in mine. His once vibrant eyes, now dulled by the relentless march of dementia, would sometimes meet mine with an eerie calmness that would send a chill down my spine. Yet, it was during these quiet, intimate moments that I found an unusual source of comfort and strength – spirituality.

Now, before we delve deeper, let me make it clear – I am not here to preach or impose any religious beliefs on you. Spirituality, as I understand it, is not confined to religious practices, and it certainly doesn't discriminate based on faith or the lack thereof. It's a deeply personal, uniquely individual journey that offers solace, strength, and often a sense of purpose. It's about finding a connection with something beyond our physical existence, and it's been a beacon of hope during my caregiving journey.

As I watched my father's personality slowly unravel under the unforgiving progression of dementia, I found myself grappling with emotions I had never experienced before. There was grief, of course, at the loss of the person I knew and loved, but there was also a profound sense of helplessness and isolation. I often felt like I was floundering in a vast, turbulent sea with no land in sight.

This is where faith and spirituality became my life raft.

There is a story that I recall about a man named Carlen Maddux. Carlen was a devoted husband and father who found himself thrust into the role of primary caregiver after his wife was diagnosed with early-onset Alzheimer's at age 50. He handled the caregiving responsibilities for five years, but eventually, the stress became too much to bear.

In his search for solace, he sought the counsel of various spiritual guides, including a nun, a minister, and a spiritual healer. His path was not smooth; it was fraught with trials and tribulations. But eventually, he found a sense of peace within himself, a sense of God's presence. This belief, this faith, provided him with the strength he needed to continue his caregiving journey.

Carlen's story resonates with me, and perhaps it will with you, too. It's a testament to the powerful role spirituality can play in our lives, especially when we find ourselves in situations that test our resilience and fortitude. It serves as a deep reminder that even when confronted with challenges and adversity, we have the capacity to discover inner strength and solace.

For me, integrating spirituality into my daily caregiving routine involved simple practices. I found solace in reading passages from spiritual texts, meditating, spending time outdoors, and reflecting on life's blessings. I discovered that spiritual music had a profound impact on my mother. These simple practices provided both of us with a sense of calm and connectedness.

And let me tell you, the benefits of incorporating spirituality into your caregiving journey are many.

Research has shown that spirituality and religion can slow cognitive decline in older adults with dementia. It helps people cope with their disease, enhancing their quality of life. It has been found to improve physical health, reducing the risk of heart disease, hypertension, and even mortality rates.

Perhaps most importantly, it offers a powerful coping mechanism. Like Carlen Maddux, many caregivers find that their faith helps them navigate the stress and emotional demands of caregiving. It offers a renewed sense of energy and purpose, which can have a transformative effect on the person they are caring for.

Summary Box

I remember sitting with my mother one sunny afternoon just a few months before she passed away. We were in her favorite spot in the garden, where the roses were in full bloom, painting the air with their sweet scent. She looked at me, and there was a flicker of recognition in her eyes. A moment of clarity that was becoming more and more rare in those days. She turned to me and said, "Life is a journey, my love, and every journey has its purpose."

At that moment, I couldn't fully grasp the depth of her words. But, as I embarked on my journey of caregiving, those words became my guiding light. They offered me comfort during the hardest days and encouraged me to find the positive aspects of dementia caregiving.

Let me share some of these insights with you, hoping they can bring you the same comfort and guidance they did for me.

Segue:

In the time before the pandemic, caring for a loved one with dementia was already a formidable task. The system wasn't perfect, and sometimes it felt like an uphill battle. But we had our routines. We had strategies to manage daily tasks, and we had a support system in place. We had connections, face-to-face interactions, and the ability to share our burdens with others. There were simple joys, too, like going for a walk in the park, visiting the local café, or just enjoying the company of friends and family.

Then came the pandemic, and everything changed. Isolation became a double-edged sword. On one side, it protected our loved ones from the virus, but on the other side, it severed the ties we had with the outside world. It was a challenging time. But even in this period of intense hardship, there were moments of unexpected beauty. I found deeper connections with my loved ones, and even when their memories were fading, our bond remained unbroken. We learned to appreciate the smaller things in life - the warmth of a shared smile, the comfort of a familiar song, the tranquility of a quiet afternoon.

Now, as we navigate the post-pandemic world, we carry these experiences with us. We are more resilient, more adaptable, and more aware of our strengths than ever before.

Embracing a mind-body-spirit approach to dementia care has been a game-changer for me. This holistic perspective goes beyond the physical aspects of caregiving and dives into the emotional and spiritual realms. It's about caring for the whole person and, in doing so, caring for ourselves.

Mindfulness, for instance, has been a lifeline. It's a practice that encourages us to stay present, to focus on the here and now rather than getting lost in the past or worrying about the future. There are various ways to practice mindfulness, and I've found a few that work well for me.

There's mindfulness meditation, where I sit quietly and focus on my breath. It's a moment of calm in the storm, a chance to center myself. There's also concentrative meditation, which I sometimes do with my loved one. We focus on a single point, like the flicker of a candle or the rhythm of a song. It's a shared experience, a moment of connection.

Positive affirmations, too, have been a powerful tool. They help me foster a positive mindset and remind me of my strength and resilience. Physical meditation, like yoga or tai chi, has been beneficial, not just for my body, but for my mind as well. And mental imagery, where I envision a peaceful scene or a happy memory, has been a source of comfort and relaxation.

Chapter 7:
Nine Practical Strategies for Supporting Your Loved One

"It isn't what we say or think that defines us, but what we do." — Jane Austen

Create a Safe and Supportive Environment for Your Loved One.

I can't help but recall the day I walked into my parents' home, both of whom were suffering from dementia. The once lively house now had a quietness about it, a stillness that seemed to seep into every corner. The people who lived there, my parents, had been transformed into mere shadows of the vibrant personalities they once were. And this house, filled with memories and laughter, was now a labyrinth of confusion and uncertainty for them.

Looking back, I realize how unprepared I was to create a safe and supportive environment for my loved ones. I wish I had the knowledge then that I have now, and it's my earnest hope to share that with you, to save you from the heartache and confusion that can accompany such a journey.

Let's begin with the basic principles of dementia caregiving. Dementia is indeed an umbrella term encompassing various conditions that impact the brain. The symptoms associated with dementia can vary but commonly include memory loss, confusion, changes in personality or behavior, and challenges with performing daily tasks. But remember, dementia does not define your loved one; they are so much more than their diagnosis. Caring for someone with dementia requires compassion, patience, and understanding. It's about preserving their dignity and creating moments of joy and connection, even in the face of such a challenging condition.

It's equally important to note that dementia can bring about behavioral and psychological symptoms, often referred to as BPSD. These can manifest as agitation, aggression, wandering, depression, or hallucinations, among other things. I remember my mother, once a calm and composed woman, growing increasingly agitated and restless.

There were times when she would not recognize me, her eyes filled with fear and confusion. It was heartbreaking, but I learned not to take it personally. Rather, I learned to approach these behaviors with empathy, understanding that they were caused by her illness, not a reflection of her feelings toward me.

Strategies for managing these symptoms can vary based on their severity and the individual's unique needs. For instance, my father, who was always a social butterfly, became increasingly withdrawn and quiet. Rather than force him into social situations that made him uncomfortable, we found solace in the quiet moments, often just sitting together in his favorite chair, watching the birds in the garden.

Recognizing and dealing with common dementia-associated behaviors can be challenging. There will be both good days and bad days. I recall days when my mother would become fixated on a particular thought or action, repeating it over and over again. It was during these times I found distraction to be a useful tool. Simply introducing a new activity or topic of conversation could help break the cycle and alleviate her distress.

Handling troubling behavior is perhaps one of the toughest aspects of caregiving. There were nights when my father would wake up disoriented, believing he was back in his childhood home, growing increasingly distressed when reality did not match his perception. In such moments, I found that validating his feelings, rather than correcting his misunderstandings, was the most compassionate approach.

Finally, creating a dementia-friendly environment is crucial. This means making necessary adaptations to the home to ensure safety and comfort. This could involve removing tripping hazards, installing safety locks, and ensuring good lighting. But it also means creating an environment of emotional safety and comfort where your loved one feels loved, valued, and understood.

Learn as Much as You Can About Your Loved One's Specific Type of Dementia and How it Affects Them

Remember my next-door neighbor, a kind elderly gentleman who had been like family to us, was diagnosed with dementia. I recall one evening when he came knocking on our door, confused and scared, unable to remember his way back home. It was that very moment, the look of fear in his eyes, that pushed me towards learning more about this disease that had begun to steal the essence of a person I held dear.

My journey into the labyrinth of dementia began that day, and I wish to share my insights and learnings with you in hopes of illuminating your path.

Dementia is a multifaceted disease, presenting in various forms and affecting every individual differently. It's not a one-size-fits-all situation, and that's why it's so crucial for you, as a caregiver, to learn as much as you can about your loved one's specific type of dementia and how it affects them.

To understand dementia, we need to delve into the various types of dementia and their symptoms. From Alzheimer's disease, the most common form, to Vascular Dementia, Lewy Body Dementia, Frontotemporal Dementia, and others, each type presents with unique characteristics and symptoms. For instance, while memory loss is a common symptom of Alzheimer's, personality changes might be more prominent in Frontotemporal Dementia.

Understanding these differences helped me immensely. I remember when my father's demeanor began to change, he became gentle, quite the opposite of his usual assertive self. Knowing that this was a manifestation of his dementia and not a deliberate change in attitude made it easier for me to adapt and provide the care he needed.

It's equally important to identify your loved one's strengths and abilities in order to create personalized care approaches. Despite the hurdles dementia presents, remember that your loved one still possesses a host of abilities, and recognizing these can make a world of difference. For example, my mother, even in the midst of her dementia journey, never lost her love for music. So, singing old songs together became a shared activity that brought us both joy and comfort.

Next, we need to understand the causes and risk factors of dementia. It is important to understand that while age is a significant risk factor for developing dementia, dementia itself is not a normal part of the aging process. Other factors like genetics, lifestyle, and certain medical conditions can also play a role. Knowledge of these can be empowering, giving you the tools to make informed decisions about your loved one's care.

When it comes to the diagnosis and progression of dementia, it's essential to remember that it's a gradual process. The disease progresses through various stages, each presenting different challenges and requiring different care strategies. My mother's condition, for instance, began with forgetfulness and gradually progressed to more severe symptoms like personality changes and difficulties with daily activities.

This brings us to the stages of dementia. There's often debate about how important these stages are. From my personal experience, I can tell you that understanding these stages can provide a roadmap of what to expect. But remember, this is just a guide. Your loved one's journey may not follow this path exactly. Despite the stages my parents went through, there were moments of clarity and connection that transcended the bounds of their disease. These were the moments I cherished the most.

Navigating the maze of dementia is a journey filled with challenges. Still, it is also a journey of deep love, resilience, and understanding. My hope is that I can provide you with the knowledge and tools to traverse this journey with your loved one, creating moments of joy and connection along the way.

Remember, you are not alone on this path.

Communicate Effectively and Compassionately with Your Loved One

One of my favorite quotes from my journey as a caregiver comes from Professor Marshall Rosenberg, the author of Nonviolent Communication. He once said, "Compassion is our innate desire to enrich another person's life." This idea resonated deeply with me and became a cornerstone of my approach to communicating with my loved ones suffering from dementia. It's not just about talking to the patient; it's about connecting heart-to-heart with compassion.

Reflecting on this idea, I'd like to share some insights and experiences from my journey, hoping they might light up yours.

In my experience, the cornerstone of any effective communication with a loved one with dementia is compassion. It's a simple word, but it holds within itself an ocean of empathy, understanding, and patience. It's about seeing beyond their current state and recognizing the person they once were, the person they still are beneath the layers of confusion and memory loss. It's about remembering that their actions and words are not deliberate defiance to upset you but rather a manifestation of a disease they did not choose to have.

When my mother's dementia advanced, she often forgot who I was. She would lash out, frightened and confused. It hurt seeing my loving mother not recognize me. But then I remembered it was the disease, not her. She wasn't deliberately trying to upset me. This understanding, this compassion, allowed me to respond with patience and love, even in the most challenging moments.

And then there's forgiveness. You see, when you're caring for your parents, old wounds might resurface. Maybe they were too rigid when you were a child, or perhaps they didn't give you the emotional support you craved. It's crucial to forgive them for their parenting so you can be the best caregiver. I had to learn this the hard way. My father was a stern man, and our relationship wasn't always smooth. But as his caregiver, I had to let go of the past, forgive him, and focus on providing the care he needed in the present.

One of the strategies I found particularly useful was changing negative labels to compassionate descriptions. The healthcare system often labels people with dementia as 'The Dementias,' 'The Wanderers,' or 'The Sundowners.' Such labels dehumanize them, reducing them to their symptoms. Instead, I would always remind myself that they are 'People living with dementia,' individuals with their unique experiences, feelings, and histories.

In my interactions with my loved ones, I tried to tune into their feelings and emotions. I listened with my heart, seeking clarification for any upsetting or challenging behavior. I tried to step into their shoes to understand their unmet needs and fears. Sometimes, it was as simple as needing reassurance, a gentle touch, or a familiar song to soothe their anxieties.

And let's not forget the power of non-verbal communication. Words might become confusing, misleading, or even scary for someone with dementia. But a comforting smile, a gentle touch, or a calm presence can communicate volumes. It can provide reassurance, convey love, and create a connection that words sometimes fail to establish.

Maintain a Routine to Help Your Loved One Feel More Secure and Comfortable

As your loved one's caregiver, you have a vast responsibility. Yet, amid the confusion and uncertainty that dementia often brings, establishing a daily routine can be a beacon of light for both of you. It may seem daunting at first, but bear with me as I guide you through this process.

Imagine the day as an unpainted canvas. It's up to you to fill it with colors and patterns that bring joy and purpose to your loved one's life while also preserving your own sanity and well-being. This is where a Daily Care Plan comes into play, providing structure and predictability in an often-unpredictable situation.

The first step in creating this plan is to reflect on the person living with dementia. Consider their likes, dislikes, strengths, abilities, and interests. Remember who they were before dementia and incorporate elements of that into their day. My mother, for instance, had a passion for gardening. So, we spent a part of our day tending to plants, which not only kept her engaged but also reminded her of the joy she found in nature.

Next, consider the daily rhythms that once existed in your loved one's life. My father was an early riser and loved to start his day with a warm cup of coffee and the morning newspaper. Even though dementia had taken a toll on his ability to comprehend the news, maintaining this routine provided a sense of comfort and familiarity.

Also consider the times of the day when your loved one is at their best. Plan the most engaging activities during these hours, ensuring you have ample time for meals, personal care, and rest. Regular wake-up and bedtime routines are equally crucial, especially if your loved one experiences sleep issues or sundowning.

A Daily Care Plan should be flexible and capable of adapting to spontaneous activities. Remember, the goal is not to have a strict timetable but rather to create a comforting rhythm that guides you through the day.

As Alzheimer's progresses, the abilities of a person with dementia will change. This is where your creativity, flexibility, and problem-solving skills will be your greatest assets. You will find yourself continuously exploring, experimenting, and adjusting your daily routine to support these changes.

Now, let's talk about the kinds of activities you can include in your daily care plan. Household chores, creative activities like art, music, or crafts, intellectual stimulation through reading or puzzles, physical activities, social interaction, and spiritual practices can all find a place in your routine.

When my mother's cognitive abilities declined, she found solace in music. We would often sit together, listening to her favorite songs. At times, she would hum along or tap her feet, and on good days, she would sing. These moments, though fleeting, were priceless.

Finally, when writing your plan, reflect on what activities work best and which don't. Be ready to adjust based on the day-to-day fluctuations in your loved one's abilities and mood. Remember, there is no need to fill every minute of the day with an activity. Balance is key. Your loved one needs both activity and rest, perhaps more frequent breaks, and varied tasks than before.

Find Joy in Small Pleasures with Your Loved by Focusing on Present Moments

In the depths of the pandemic, we were pushed to the limit, weren't we? Yet, in the midst of it all, many of us discovered silver linings. Families found new ways to connect, spending more time together over shared meals or movie nights. We learned to appreciate the little things that we often took for granted – the sound of laughter, the comforting smell of a home-cooked meal, and the warmth of a shared blanket. For caregivers, gratitude might have come in the form of technology bridging the gap of physical distance, allowing us to "see" our loved ones even in isolation.

Gratitude has been called our "social glue." It's a fundamental part of what makes us human, allowing us to create connections and strengthen our relationships. It can lift us up from the depths of despair, reminding us of the good in our lives and the world around us.

In my journey as a caregiver, I found that focusing on gratitude didn't mean ignoring the pain or difficulties. Instead, it allowed me to see them in a different light. When my mother's dementia took away her personality, the woman I had known and loved all my life, I was devastated. But amidst that heartbreak, I found moments of gratitude. I was grateful for the years we'd had together, for the love she'd given me, and for the strength I found in myself to care for her.

Gratitude is a lot more than just an emotion. It's a practice, a mindset, and even a lifestyle. Researchers, Robert Emmons and Michael McCullough define gratitude as "recognizing one has experienced a positive outcome and that there was an external source for this positive outcome."

Adopting an attitude of gratitude can have powerful impacts on our health and well-being. It can amplify the good in our lives, rescue us from toxic feelings, and strengthen our relationships. Research over the last 20 years has shown that practicing gratitude can lead to better sleep, increased physical activity, healthier behaviors, and even fewer aches and pains.

Take Care of Yourself as a Caregiver and Seek Support from Others

"Sometimes, the one who flies the plane must remember to put on their own oxygen mask before helping others." This quote has always resonated with me, and it couldn't be more accurate for us caregivers. Navigating through the maze of dementia is indeed like flying a plane in turbulent weather. It's a journey filled with unexpected challenges, heartache, and, often, a profound sense of isolation. But my dear reader, it's crucial to remember that you can't take care of your loved one if you don't take care of yourself first.

Be a Healthy Caregiver

It's not uncommon for a caregiver to feel so overwhelmed with responsibilities that you neglect your own well-being. I've been there myself. However, the most valuable thing you can do for your loved one is to stay physically and emotionally strong.

See the Doctor

I know how tempting it is to try to do everything by yourself. I've walked that road, trying to juggle multiple roles, only to end up exhausted and stressed. But please, don't do it alone. Seek support from family, friends, your faith community, and organizations like the Alzheimer's Association®.

Ensure to see your physician regularly—at least annually—and listen to what your body tells you. Don't shrug off signs like exhaustion, stress, sleeplessness, or changes in appetite or behavior. I remember dismissing my persistent fatigue as just part and parcel of caregiving, only to be diagnosed with adrenal fatigue later. These symptoms are your body's warning signs and ignoring them can lead to a serious decline in your physical and mental health.

If you're caring for someone in the late stages of Alzheimer's, it's essential to talk to your healthcare provider about the seasonal flu shot. Getting vaccinated not only protects you, but also safeguards the person you're caring for.

Get Moving

Exercise is a crucial part of staying healthy. Not only does it help relieve stress and prevent diseases, but it also makes you feel good. I've found my morning yoga routine to be my haven of calm amidst the storm. But with the constant demands of caregiving, finding the time to exercise often feels like an uphill battle.

Here are some strategies that worked for me:

- *Accept help:* Don't hesitate to take up offers from friends and family members to watch over your loved one while you exercise.

- *Start small:* While the recommended exercise routine is 30 minutes of physical activity at least five days a week, even 10 minutes a day can make a difference. Fit in what you can, and gradually work towards your goal.

- *Find something you love:* When exercise becomes a joy rather than a chore, it's easier to incorporate it into your routine. For me, it's yoga. For you, it could be a brisk walk in the park or a dance class.

Exercising with your loved one can also be a great bonding activity. My dad and I used to take short walks in our neighborhood. Even when his memory faded, he always seemed to remember our little adventures.

Eat Well

Eating a balanced, heart-healthy diet not only benefits your overall health but may also help protect your brain. Consider adopting a Mediterranean diet, which emphasizes whole grains, fruits, vegetables, fish, nuts, olive oil, and other healthy fats. Involving a person with dementia in meal preparations can be a wonderful way to engage them.

Consider Professional Care Options for Your Loved One When Necessary

It was a crisp Saturday morning in my hometown when I first stepped into an adult daycare center. I had been navigating the confusing labyrinth of dementia care for my mother for almost a year, and I was feeling the toll it was taking on me. As a caregiver, it was challenging trying to balance my own needs with the needs of my mother, who had been slowly losing her memory and cognitive abilities. A friend had mentioned adult daycare to me, and I was desperate for respite, so I decided to give it a try.

Like many of you, I had never even considered adult daycare for my mother. The idea seemed foreign, and I wasn't sure what to expect. But when I walked into the bustling center, I was immediately put at ease. The staff was warm and welcoming, and the other participants, people like my mother, seemed happy and engaged. It felt like a community, and I felt a sense of relief wash over me.

Adult daycare centers play a valuable role in supporting both caregivers and individuals with dementia. These centers offer a much-needed break for caregivers, providing them with respite from their caregiving responsibilities. By promoting socialization and reducing feelings of loneliness, adult daycare centers contribute to the overall emotional and social well-being of individuals with dementia, enhancing their quality of life and sense of belonging.

Now, I know what you're thinking, "Isn't it just like a community senior center?" And the answer is no. While traditional community senior centers are great for relatively healthy older people, adult daycare centers are specially designed to care for those with physical or cognitive disabilities who need more supervision and services.

In fact, more than half of the older attendees at adult daycare facilities have cognitive impairments, like my mother. But the benefits of these centers extend beyond just providing a safe environment. A study published in the journal "The Gerontologist" found that older people who attend these centers have a better quality of life. They receive health-related, social, psychological, and behavioral benefits, particularly for those with dementia and other cognitive impairments.

Not only do these centers provide benefits for our loved ones, but they also have a positive impact on us, the caregivers. A 2021 study found that both dementia patients and caregivers slept better, with fewer disturbances, on nights before the patients attended adult daycare. Other research has shown that using adult daycare has a positive impact on caregivers' mood, health, and relationships, reducing their sense of "role overload."

When choosing an adult daycare center for your loved one with dementia, there are several factors to consider. Factors such as geographic location and range of services offered can impact the cost, which on average is around $1,690 a month, or $78 per day, according to a 2021 survey. Medicare typically does not cover the fees for adult daycare centers. However, there are other government programs that may offer financial assistance to help make adult daycare more affordable than the option of hiring a worker to provide in-home care.

Navigating the world of adult daycare during the COVID-19 pandemic presented additional challenges. Many centers had to temporarily close or limit their hours, and the disease impacted both participants and staff. But the industry adapted, with most centers implementing daily COVID-19 screenings and other safety measures. As of 2021, some areas have begun to ease certain precautions, while others have maintained measures such as mask-wearing.

One of the most important things to remember when considering adult daycare is knowing when it might be needed. The Adult Day Services Association (NADSA) recommends that caregivers explore adult daycare services when they notice certain signs in their older loved ones. These signs may include difficulties in structuring daily activities, feelings of isolation and loneliness, or experiences of anxiety or depression.

Honor Your Loved One's Dignity and Celebrate Their Life

There are moments in life that stay with you forever, like indelible ink etched into the fabric of your memory. One such moment for me was the celebration of my friend Kim's mother's life, not after her passing but while she was still with us, living with advanced dementia. I'm here to share that story with you and, hopefully, provide you with some inspiration and guidance.

Here is her story:

"My mother, Judy, was a vibrant soul. She loved life and had a clear vision of how she wanted to be remembered. She wanted her life to be celebrated, not mourned. Years ago, she told me she wished for a "life celebration," a gathering of family and friends reminiscing, laughing, and sharing stories by her lakeside home, her ashes spread over the gentle waves of the lake she loved so dearly.

"But as her dementia progressed, her savings dwindled, and we had to sell the cherished cottage to afford her care. Her world shrank to her memory care assisted living facility, a handful of friends who still visited, and the loving staff who cared for her. I was struck by the realization that the quality of her day-to-day life was what mattered most, not a celebration after her passing.

"Yet, the desire for a celebration lingered. I felt that my mother deserved a party, deserved to be the center of attention, to feel joy and love while she was still here to enjoy it.

"So, when Mom moved into a nursing home, I decided to plan a little gathering for her 74th birthday. The invitation read, "Though she's living with advanced dementia, Mom will delight in your presence. We're sharing our love and affection for her now while she can enjoy it." It was a leap of faith, an experiment in love and joy in the face of the relentless march of dementia.

"Few of Mom's family remained – her out-of-state sister, nieces, and nephews, but they came. My children were there, as were some of Mom's favorite neighbors from the lake. Two women who visited her every week also came - an aide from the memory care facility and a massage therapist who often read to Mom and took her outside. They were paid to be there, but to Mom, they were special companions, bringing a spark of joy to her life.

"I cooked the meal and baked Mom's favorite angel food cake – just like the one she used to make for my birthdays. We invited the entire nursing home staff to join us. We set out old photos of Mom and her family, and the staff came down to eat and learn more about my mother as a person.

"Throughout the party, a harpist played Mom's favorite pieces, including "Clair de Lune," filling the room with a serene, warm ambiance. Mom was quiet, but her eyes were bright. She held people's hands, smiled, and her laughter filled the room at just the right moments. It was a small, intimate gathering filled with profound love and joy.

"When Mom passed away the following year, my initial instinct was to plan another celebration. But as I looked around, I realized that those who would travel for the funeral were the same people who had already come to the birthday celebration. We had already shared what Mom had envisioned, and it felt right to say "goodbye" in a more personal way. So, my family and

I hiked down to the lake by our old cottage and gently released Mom's ashes into the water."

Summary Box

Let's take a moment to reflect on our journey together:

- We began by understanding what dementia is, stripping away the medical jargon, and understanding the condition from a human perspective. We acknowledge that dementia is not merely a medical condition but a profound change in our loved one's life and ours.

- We then delved into the emotional journey of being a caregiver, acknowledging the grief, the fear, and the sense of loss. But also, we recognized the love, resilience, and the profound bond that often blossoms in these challenging times.

- We explored the practical aspects of caregiving, from managing day-to-day tasks, ensuring the safety and comfort of our loved one, to navigating the complicated landscape of medical care and financial planning.

- We learned about communication and how to connect with our loved ones even when the traditional paths seem blocked. We discovered the power of touch, of music, of shared.

- We addressed the difficult topics of behavioral changes, of dealing with confusion, anger, and even aggression. But we learned to see beyond these behaviors, to the person we love who is still there, just beneath the surface.

- And finally, we talked about self-care and the importance of taking care of ourselves physically, emotionally, and spiritually. We acknowledged that it's okay to ask for help, to take a break, to cry, to laugh, to live.

Segue:

Each chapter of this book, each part of our journey together, links to form a chain of understanding, hope, and resilience. You've learned not just to navigate the maze of dementia care but to do so with grace, love, and a heart full of hope.

I want to congratulate you. You've walked this path, you've absorbed these lessons, and you've embraced this journey with open arms. You're not just a caregiver; you're a beacon of love and hope. Your journey doesn't end with the last page of this book. It continues each day, with each smile, each shared memory, and each moment of love and connection with your loved one.

As we end this chapter together, remember this: You are stronger than you think. You are more resilient than you believe. Most importantly, in the face of dementia, you carry within you a powerful, unending wellspring of love and hope.

Thank you for joining me on this journey. Here's to a better future, one filled with love, understanding, resilience, and hope. Remember, you are not alone, and with the lessons from this book, you're well-equipped to navigate this with grace.

Conclusion

Dementia is a battle we did not choose, but it is a battle we must face. As we wrap up this journey together through the pages of this book, I want to remind you of the key points we've discussed.

We started with understanding dementia - its types, symptoms, causes, risk factors, and progression. We discussed the emotional rollercoaster that comes with a dementia diagnosis, both for the person affected and their loved ones. We explored the importance of compassionate caregiving, navigating the rough waters of challenges and stresses, the significance of emotional connections, and the beauty of embracing this journey, despite its hardships. We concluded with nine practical strategies for supporting your loved one and maintaining their dignity and quality of life.

Remember, caring for someone with dementia can present challenges, but it is also a deeply rewarding experience. The lessons learned from this book can serve as valuable tools to enhance the care you provide and make a positive impact on your loved one's life. Applying the knowledge and insights gained from this book to your daily life can help you navigate the journey of dementia caregiving with compassion, empathy, and understanding.

Now, I want you to do two things for me.

First, I want you to remember this: You are not alone. You are part of a community of caregivers who understand, empathize, and stand beside you. Use the tools and strategies we've discussed in this book, reach out to others when you need to, and never, ever lose hope.

Second, if this book has been of help to you, I would greatly appreciate it if you could leave a review on Amazon. Your feedback will not only help me to improve, but it will also help other caregivers find this book and, hopefully, find some comfort and guidance. You can leave a review by scanning the code below.

As we conclude this journey, I want to leave you with a personal note. I understand the emotional impact dementia can have on both the person living with it and their loved ones. Throughout my journey, I've learned the importance of education, advocacy, and empathy, all of which I hope I have conveyed through this book.

I hope this book served as a resource for those affected by dementia, providing practical advice and emotional support. I also hope it fosters a greater understanding of dementia, reducing the stigma and misinformation that often accompanies it.

Thank you for accompanying me on this journey of exploration and insight. I wish you all the strength and grace as you navigate your own maze of dementia care. Remember, even in the hardest moments, there is always hope. And sometimes, that hope can come from the most unexpected places.

Take care, and good luck on your journey.

Warm regards,

G.M. Grace

Leave a Review

As an independent author with a small marketing budget, reviews are my livelihood on this platform. If you got value from this book, I'd really appreciate it if you left your honest feedback by reviewing this book on Amazon. You can do so by scanning the QR code below. I love hearing from my readers, and I personally read every single review.

Resources

Administration for Community Living Website: www.acl.gov	Meals on Wheels Website: https://www.mealsonwheelsamerica.org / Phone Number: 888-998-6325
AIDS Crisis Line Phone Number: 800-221-7044	Medicaid Website: https://www.medicaid.gov/
ALZConnected Website: www.alzconnected.org	Medicare Website: https://www.medicare.gov/
Alzheimer's Foundation of America Website: www.alzfdn.org	Memory Café Directory Website: www.memorycafedirectory.com
Alzheimer's Association Website: www.alz.org Contact: 800-272-3900	National Academy of Elder Law Attorneys Website: https://www.naela.org/ Email: naela@naela.org
American Association of Poison Control Centers Phone Number: 800-222-1222	National Adult Day Services Association Website: https://www.nadsa.org/ Toll-Free Number: 1-877-745-1440 Email: info@nadsa.org
American Council on Aging How Medicaid Can Help Seniors Cover the Cost of Assisted Living Website: https://www.medicaidplanningassistance.o rg/assisted-living/ Toll-Free Number: 1-800-677-1116 Email: eldercarelocator@n4a.org	National Alliance for Caregiving Website: www.caregiving.org Contact: 202-918-1013 Email: info@caregiving.org
Caregiver Action Network Website: www.caregiveraction.org Contact: 202-454-3970 Email: info@caregiveraction.org	National Council on Alcoholism & Drug Dependency Hope Line Phone Number: 800-622-2255

Caregiver Action Network's Family Caregiver Toolbox Website: www.caregiveraction.org/family-caregiver-toolbox Contact: 202-454-3970 Email: info@caregiveraction.org	National Crisis Line - Anorexia and Bulimia Phone Number: 800-233-4357
Center to Advance Palliative Care Website: www.getpalliativecare.org Phone Number: 212-201-2670 Email: capc@mssm.edu	National Do Not Call Registry Website: https://www.donotcall.gov/
Cleveland Clinic's Healthy Brains Website: www.healthybrains.org	National Domestic Violence Hotline Phone Number: 800-799-7233
Community Resource Finder Website: https://www.communityresourcefinder.org/	National Hopeline Network Phone Number: 800-SUICIDE (800-784-2433)
Consumer Financial Protection Bureau Website: https://www.consumerfinance.gov/	National Hospice and Palliative Care Organization Website: www.caringinfo.org Phone Number: 800-658-8898 Email: caringinfo@nhpco.org
Crisis Text Line Text 'DESERVE' TO 741-741	National Institute on Aging Website: www.nia.nih.gov
Dementia Friendly America Website: www.dfamerica.org	National Memory Screening Program Website: https://alzfdn.org/memory-screening/ Phone Number: 866-232-8484 Email: info@alzfdn.org
Education in Palliative and End-of-Life Care Website: www.epec.net Phone Number: 312-503-3732 Email: info@epec.net	National Respite Locator Service Website: www.archrespite.org/respitelocator
Eldercare Locator Website: https://eldercare.acl.gov Phone Number: 800-677-1116 Email: eldercarelocator@n4a.org	National Suicide Prevention Lifeline Phone Number: 800-273-TALK (8255)

Family Caregiver Alliance Website: www.caregiver.org Contact: 800-445-8106 Email: info@caregiver.org	NIA Alzheimer's and Related Dementias Education and Referral (ADEAR) Center Website: www.nia.nih.gov/alzheimers Phone Number: 800-438-4380 Email: adear@nia.nih.gov
Free Resources for Caregivers of People With Alzheimer's Disease and Related Dementias Website: https://www.alzheimers.gov/life- with-dementia/resources-caregivers Phone Number: 800-438-4380 Email: adear@nia.nih.gov	Self-Harm Hotline Phone Number: 800-366-8288
GLBT Hotline Phone Number: 888-843-4564	TransLifeline Website: https://www.translifeline.org Phone Number: 877-565-8860
Headspace Website: https://www.headspace.com/ Email: help@headspace.com	TREVOR Crisis Hotline Phone Number: 866-488-7386
Hospice Foundation of America Website: www.hospicefoundation.org Phone Number: 800-854-3402 Email: info@hospicefoundation.org	U.S. Department of Veterans Affairs Website: www.va.gov Toll-free number: 1-800-827-1000 TTY: 1-800-829-4833
Insight Timer Website: https://insighttimer.com/	Veterans Crisis Line Website: https://www.veteranscrisisline.net
International End of Life Doula Association Website: https://inelda.org/ Phone Number: 201-540-9049 Email: info@inelda.org	Visiting Nurse Associations of America Website: www.vnaa.org Phone Number: 888-866-8773 Email: vnaa@vnaa.org
Lifeline Crisis Chat Website: https://suicidepreventionlifeline.org/chat/ (Online live messaging)	Well Spouse Association Website: www.wellspouse.org Phone Number: 800-838-0879 Email: info@wellspouse.org

| Managing Money: A Caregiver's Guide to Finance Website: https://www.alz.org/media/wi/documents/ Day-1-Keynote-3-Managing-Money-Participants-Guide.pdf | |

Index

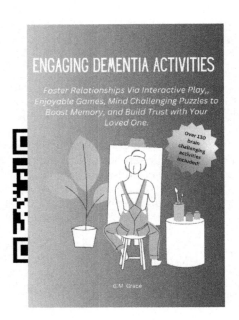

More Books by G.M. Grace

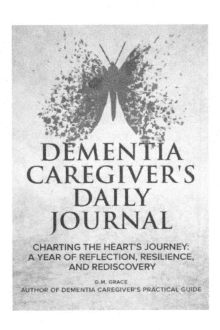

Printed in Great Britain
by Amazon